JUST MISSED HARLEY STREET
Memories of a General Practitioner

By

James Carne

Grosvenor House
Publishing Limited

The right of James Carne to be identified as the author of this
work has been asserted by him in accordance with Section 78
of the Copyright, Designs and Patents Act 1988

The book cover picture is copyright to Inmagine Corp LLC

This book is published by
Grosvenor House Publishing Ltd
28-30 High Street, Guildford, Surrey, GU1 3EL.
www.grosvenorhousepublishing.co.uk

A CIP record for this book
is available from the British Library

ISBN 978-1-78148-849-2

Dedicated to Cleo, and any other great-grandchildren still to come, in the hope that when they are old enough to read it, they will find it interesting.

About the Author

James Carne was born in London and has lived there most of his life. He qualified as a doctor in 1952, at a time when the National Health Service was emerging as a major force, and, after a period in the RAF, practiced in Hackney, London, for over 40 years. He was a part time academic in the Department of General Practice at St Bartholomew's Hospital, and Queen Mary College, London. He is also a Fellow of the Expert Witness Institute and Member of the Chartered Institute of Arbitrators.

CONTENTS

Contents

CHAPTER I

Introduction

Life is a sandwich. Not exactly a club sandwich, and not, as the old Rabbi joke informs us, a bowl of cherries. I started writing this journal as a blog in July 2008, being helped in setting it up by my number three grandson, Alex. By August of the following year I gave myself a sabbatical of a few months until December 2009 when I found a new enthusiasm and was advised by my number one grandson, Tom, who is a professional journalist, to divide the contents into three portions: hence the concept of a sandwich was born. The slices of bread are represented by the ending and starting of life and the filling by the in-between professional life I was privileged to lead. I am reminded that it was Shakespeare who wrote that in the seven ages of man, all the world was just a stage in which each of us plays many parts. I am also reminded of another great writer, Anthony Trollope, who described the period in which I now find myself as "the brown leaf period of life".

Nine months after I started writing I realised it was no longer a blog in the true sense of the word, but more an attempt at an autobiography, or if not exactly an autobiography, a stroll through my life and experiences. As portions were written, I remembered experiences I thought had been long forgotten.

Finding a title for the book has proved challenging. The book is not an autobiography, but more an accumulation of memories, observations, anecdotes and 'bon mots' that have made up at least a portion of my life. Although from first deciding that a doctor was what I wanted to be, I always envisaged this would be in general practice; and so it turned out. A passing remark from a patient many years ago, summed up the way I felt, and hence the title "Just Missed Harley Street".

Writing has set me thinking about growing old and what it might mean to an individual. In the summer of 2008, the *Times* printed an obituary of Professor Janet Askham, sociologist and gerontologist. Although not known to me previously, I noted that it quotes from her as saying that "ageing is both a social and biological phenomenon: one can start with the notion of when old age begins. There is no biological starting point: it is socially determined. People become old because they are defined as old – by the attitudes and behaviour of others and by laws, rules or policies." Maybe because she died at a relatively young age, 66, Professor Askham missed an important point, the insight for which only comes with greater personal experience. Being old also depends on the perception one has of oneself: others only reflect what one displays. I cannot be alone in regretting that in my head, life is a bed of roses but my body is not always in agreement. Nevertheless, for generations people have grown old at the point they conceive themselves to be old. Numerical age has nothing to do with it, but actionable age has. An old Jewish joke puts it rather succinctly. An old man complains to his doctor that "up there it is always *Simchas Torah* (rejoicing of the Law) but down there it is usually *Yom Kippur* (day of Atonement)".

Over the years I have contemplated the question: "When does one first feel old?" It is many years since policemen looked old, to be replaced by Greek Orthodox Priests and other religious men. Now everyone seems to look young, so I have to rely on other examples. It was not good when a younger person first offered me a seat on the bus, and even less reassuring the first time I accepted. Now, occasionally, even old people offer me their seat . . . What else? Sitting on a committee with a group of distinguished professional people and realising you are no longer the young pretender, but the oldest one present. Being irritated by people deliberately speaking louder (and slower) because they assume you must be hard of hearing – and then finding yourself asking people to speak up because you really are. I will omit all the obvious anecdotes beloved of comedians: "Bending down to tie your shoelaces and forgetting why you are there"; "Pausing for breath half way up the stairs and forgetting whether you were on the way down or up". I am sure there are many more. I suppose one truly knows one is getting old when a fear of falling sets in. I remember an old teacher of mine (a neurologist) stating this in a lecture and being greeted with collective disbelief. Time has proven him right, and increasing awareness of my contemporaries has confirmed the accuracy of the observation.

CHAPTER II

The 1930s

If asked what was the most memorable experience of the year 1928, most people would reply that it was the start of the recession that turned into depression a few months into 1929. From a personal point of view, I would have to answer that it was the year I first appeared to the world, blissfully unaware of the impending financial disaster.

At the start of the 1930s I was not yet two years old. My life was fairly routine for a middle class child growing up in that decade. Although not rich my father, who worked as a bank executive, had his income augmented a little by my mother who had her own small (and not always successful) millinery business. I have since estimated that we lived on an income of about £500 a year, but this was enough in those days to afford both a living-in maid and a nanny to look after three siblings and myself. I was the youngest, and inevitably I was spoiled either in reality, or in the imagination of my older brother and sisters. I think our nanny did have a soft spot for me, and certainly this was returned in no small measure. Elizabeth (not her real name) joined our family when she was only about fourteen and stayed until she married her childhood sweetheart; I was six. We remained in contact and I have warm memories of being allowed to stay with her from time to time. Her new husband, a carpenter by trade, was called up when war was declared and served throughout in the navy. On demobilisation my mother helped him find a job with a firm of builders, who expanded into property development and later offered him a partnership in their thriving business. As a result he finished up a very rich man. It is many years since I last saw Elizabeth, and by that time I had reached adulthood, was a practising doctor and was pleased to find that Elizabeth was living a comfortable rural life with children of her own. I think I did, however, suffer a twinge of jealousy when I realised that her own children meant more to her than I did!

Rabbi Schonfield had opened what was probably one of the first wholly Jewish faith schools, with religious education a priority. For some reason my parents felt the need to support this venture, and in consequence I was sent there as my first experience of organised learning, at the age of five. The experiment only lasted a year after which, for reasons never explained to me, I was transferred to a small private school where my brother was already a pupil. The headmaster owned the school and was a fiery, rather eccentric man who seemed to take a delight in striding round the corridors of the school in trousers that were just too short, so the space between turn ups and shoes always showed a large flash of multi-coloured sock. He lived in the same road as us and had two daughters who were our contemporaries and friends of my older sisters. Although not close friends with the family, it did seem to diminish any fear of him we might otherwise have had.

Freed from the shackles of a religious school, I found I had a certain expertise in games, especially those involving bat and a moving ball, and my energies henceforth were about equally divided between academia and sports. Cricket was my favourite game and although it was superseded by tennis in later years, cricket still maintains a high place among my interests. I remember an occasion when I was about eight, being put in to bat and sometime later was still batting, while all the others were impatiently awaiting their turn. It required the master coming on to bowl to eventually get rid of me. On another occasion there was a game scheduled to be played and to my dismay I had been given a detention (for what, I have long since forgotten). I had the bright notion of asking the headmaster if instead of the detention I had been given, I could suffer "the slipper" – actually a utensil applied to one's bottom, used when the headmaster didn't feel strokes from the more painful cane were justified. He agreed to my proposal, thus freeing me to be able to play my beloved game, but I think he felt I had shown some courage and responded by giving me very light taps, which I barely felt. ("Barely", I hasten to add, relating to the feeling, not to the part of my body to which the slipper was applied . . .) This was a mistake, since although it was my first taste of corporal punishment, I thought it a doddle and something not to be feared. A few weeks later, the headmaster, who was rather eccentric and had spy holes built into the classroom doors so he could secretly observe the behaviour of a class without being seen himself, caught me through this device, surreptitiously kicking the boy seated in front of me. To my horror the door was thrown open and my name called out; I was instructed to attend his study during break. On this occasion he had no sympathetic or secret admiration for my actions, and I received six strokes of the cane. It hurt – a lot. At least it was successful in teaching me two lessons. I have never since risked a repeat performance of the cane, and I learned to be very wary of volunteering for an alternative punishment in the future.

In my second or third year at the school, two new faces appeared and we were asked to take them under our wing even though they spoke very little English. It turned out they were refugees from the Civil War in Spain, which at that time was at its height. At that age war, especially if it was being fought at some distant place, was not something to which one gave a lot of thought, but their presence at the school was the first experience I had of hearing about some of the horrors associated with fighting. I believe they were (or at least their parents were) Republican and anti-Franco. They quickly became assimilated in the school, and rapidly learned to speak English, but I do not know what became of them, or what horrific experiences they or their families might have suffered.

In 1934 my parents discovered a farm in a small village near Braintree in Essex, where the wife of the farmer catered for up to about twenty children during the summer holidays. For the next four or five years, my siblings and I were dispatched to the farm for about six weeks during the school summer holidays. By today's standards, with children often accompanying their parents on holiday, this may sound harsh, but in fact we had great fun. To call it a farm is perhaps rather too ambitious. The farmhouse was large enough to accommodate us all in comfort, and the grounds were huge – or looked it, to our tiny eyes. There were two cows to provide us all with fresh full cream milk. I remember the cream lay like a golden yellow band on the top of the snow-coloured milk and there was always a rush to be the first to obtain it. At times we drank the milk still warm from the cow. (Later, as a doctor, I would realise we were fortunate that the milk was not infected with the tubercle bacillus, although it is possible this was where I acquired the useful protection against TB as shown by a positive mantoux test, taken when I became a medical student.) The only other farmyard animals in residence were numerous chickens, which supplied us with all the eggs we could eat, and I think a couple of pigs to eat up the left over food and scraps.

We sometimes visited neighbouring farms and during harvest time considered it a great treat to be allowed to sit on the tractor while the farmer drove round his land. Combine harvesters were a new novelty and one watched in wonderment as they ploughed through the ripened crop in neighbouring wheat fields, spewing out the rubbish and leaving cartfuls of the wheat germ intact. Haystacks were scattered round the area and made ideal places to play on and slide down; there was one dreadful occasion when my sister mistook a manure heap for a haystack and made an awful mess of her clothes. Carthorses could be ridden from their overnight sojourn in the outer fields, back to their places of heavy work. On one occasion I was perched on one of the apparently passive horses when he decided to canter instead of walking sedately. To an eight year old boy this was very frightening and inevitably I fell off. Fortunately no real damage was done, but it was very painful. I haven't sat on a horse since.

These memories are all real, but one memory has been lost in the course of time: it never seemed to rain and if it did I cannot for the life of me remember how we occupied ourselves. But of course it is universally acknowledged that when one thinks back on holidays, it is always sunny. A special treat was to walk half a mile down the lane to the sweet shop where a dear old lady – she must have been about forty, old to me – served us with sherbet dabs, aniseed balls, pontefract cakes and, if we could get them into our mouths, gob stoppers. The local blacksmith, just a short walk down the road, was also often visited: his skilful shoeing of farm horses and metal craftwork was a constant delight.

The farm also housed a tennis court, putting green and croquet lawn. Being sporty I was in my element and there was always someone to play with. One year, a young boy from France was a guest and he introduced us to a game we called "kiki peg". It was a combination of hide and seek and touch; a lot of fun. I also learned a lesson during these vacations, which I have carried through life. I was about nine, and had just been introduced to the joys of tennis. Another guest was a much older man of about twenty-five. Seeing him on his own one day, I asked him if he would like to play a game of tennis. Cheeky – but rather to my surprise he accepted the invitation, asking me to wait while he got ready for the game. To my even greater surprise, he came down the stairs about ten minutes later, clad completely in whites (long trousers of course) as if he was about to enter the tournament at Wimbledon. Not surprisingly I got thrashed. Still, the degree of respect a twenty-five-year-old man showed for a nine-year-old boy taught me something about respect I hope I have not forgotten.

During our time at the farm in the summer of 1938, two important events of worldwide significance occurred. First, the crisis threatening war with Germany and Neville Chamberlain's historic declaration of "peace in our time". Second – and what at the time I thought much more significant – Len Hutton's record score of 364 in the test match against Australia. Even in the absence of TV, listening to the radio as these historic occasions were described was exciting. Although TV was not a facility available at the farm, it had recently been invented and a few people did possess one. In the late 1930s, friends of my parents, who were in the film business, had opened a cinema in Kilburn, which was billed as the largest in Europe. Apart from showing two films and a stage show plus news and cartoons (all in one sitting!) it also boasted a large restaurant where one could eat lunch, tea or dinner before or after the film. As an added attraction, a television had been placed in the middle of the restaurant so any diners present could watch "this modern miracle of technology". The screen size was no more than about twelve by twelve inches, and of course the image was black and white. Nevertheless, I felt very privileged when, as friends of the cinema owner, we were invited to watch the FA Cup final, the first year in which it was televised. Previously one had to be content with radio commentary, and to help follow the game, the Radio Times printed a picture of the football pitch divided up into numbered squares or grids, rather like a road map is nowadays. As the commentator described the match a voice in the background would intone, "square B5" or "square C3" and you would see where the ball was positioned. The commentary was related with increasingly breathless excitement, as exemplified by the famous George Allison, who doubled up as manager of Arsenal football club, and his excited description of "It's a goal, it's a goal – oh no it isn't!" became his catchphrase. (Perhaps things have not changed that much: the other day I heard a radio commentator discuss a near-goal by saying "what a goal that would have been if only he had scored".) To return to the first TV football game I watched, imagine the scene: a twelve inch screen, black and white and sitting in a large restaurant; tiny blurred figures running around what in effect was a tiny, colourless pitch; and yet the excitement I felt then still lives with me now.

During these years, even at my young age, I was well aware of the threat of fascism and the menace it held for so many of us. My father would take my brother and I to Speakers' Corner in Hyde Park or occasionally a similar forum in Finsbury Park. I remember the loathing and filth poured out by the fascist followers of Oswald Moseley. At the age of nine I found it very difficult to understand why I was so hated just because of my religion, something over which I had no control. Now, over 80, I still find it incomprehensible. Such prejudices are still present, of course, ethnic origin joining religion as one of those things for which you can be hated for being *who* you are, rather than *what* you are. In such ways has the world progressed!

The threat of what might happen if Hitler had his way and conquered Britain was ever-present during the late 1930s. Although aware of the horrors of people – my people – being rounded up and sent to concentration camps, I cannot remember feeling any fear that it might actually happen to me. I have a vivid memory of a client of my father, who made trips to England from Germany every few months, each time smuggling in money and jewellery, which he would deposit in the bank where my father worked. On one occasion he was invited to our house for dinner, and I remember this very pleasant man with a fund of stories to tell, some of which were really very frightening. Sadly he returned to Germany one time too many, and we never heard of him again.

The shadows of war returned during 1939, just one year after Chamberlain's "peace in our time" speech, and became a reality on the 3 September. War was finally declared.

CHAPTER III

World War II and Evacuation

The crisis in August and September 1938 had prepared us for what to expect in 1939, when "peace in our time" turned to "war in our time". As in 1938, when news of the increasing threat of war emerged in 1939 we were at the farm where we spent our summer holidays. I think we believed that the pattern would be repeated: Chamberlain would alight from his plane with another piece of paper in his hand, and we would all return to school. This time it was different: we had to return home from the farm earlier than planned and on arriving home we were informed by our parents that they had decided all of us, except my eldest sister who had already left school, should be evacuated to the country, where we would be safer from the bombing and, presumably, from the threat of invasion. All three of us that were involved were at different schools: my sister was at a girls' grammar school, my brother at a co-educational grammar school and I was still at junior primary school, with another year to go before hopefully joining my brother at grammar school. All three schools were in Willesden, North West London, where we were living since moving from Stamford Hill in 1936. In their wisdom, and quite rightly, my parents felt it would be best if we were not split up, so had opted for us all to be evacuated with my sister's girls' school. Where we would end up, or when we would actually travel were unknown factors, so for the week before war was declared, we found ourselves packed and ready to go whenever and wherever the fates decided. Each day we would arrive at my sister's school to spend the day at various activities arranged by the teachers, and would then return home in the evening if nothing had happened. It was all really quite good fun, and being a ten-year-old boy among a whole bevy of girls ranging in age from eleven to eighteen, and of varying nubility, I think I was really quite spoiled, and can certainly remember enjoying all the attention I was receiving.

On the fourth day of this regime, things became rather more serious and we were informed that "today is likely to be the day we were to go away". I believe my memory is correct that it was on Friday 1 September 1939 that we started on our travels, and we divided up into groups and marched in crocodile fashion to the bus that was to take us to Euston Station, from where, it was rumoured, we were going to Northampton, a Midlands town about 60 miles from London. However, it did not quite turn out like this. The three of us, although still together, were in a group that was behind the others, and as their train filled up, there was no room for our group and we were told that we would be on the next train going only as far as Luton. Fortunately the mistress in charge of our group was having nothing of it! She was not going to let her "girls" become separated from their fellow pupils, with the risk of finishing up at a different school. I can still remember her rampant voice in true Miss Jean Brodie style arguing with the stationmaster that arrangements had been made for the "whole school" to go to Northampton, and if it was the last thing she was going to do, she would see to it that we would finish up there as well. Rather surprisingly, considering all the circumstances of an inevitable war, and hundreds of thousands of children being evacuated within a few days of each other, she was successful and although I do not remember whether we waited for a later train or changed at Luton, we finished up in Northampton, rather later than the rest of the school and very tired, but at least the whole school had remained intact. As luck and fate would have it, we later discovered that my brother's school and my school had also finished up in Northampton, so we were all able to attend our own schools, and a year later, having passed the scholarship (now a dirty word, but at the time considered an achievement), I was able to transfer to the grammar school where my brother already attended. In fact, when things were eventually sorted out, my sister's all girl school joined up with the girls of my brother's co-educational school, and the boys from the mixed school joined up with boys from an all boys grammar school from the same area of London. We were then accommodated at separate senior schools in Northampton, using the premises for half a day while our hosts used them for the rest of the day. I cannot speak for the girls' school, but the local boys' school was very smart with the pupils wearing boaters when walking in the town: it also had fine playing fields attached at the rear of the premises, with a famous large private mental hospital bordering the school. It was really more like a public school than a grammar school, and we benefited accordingly.

Because we were only at school for half a day, the authorities had to make arrangements to keep us out of mischief for the other half. In our case one of the masters took over a large, but empty, house and with the help of some of the sixth formers (some of whom were very soon to go to serve in the "real war", and a few of whom did not return), set up what they called "The Youth Hostel". Organised activities kept us busy and further friendships were made. I have no doubt it contributed enormously to our feelings of security in the very artificial state in which we found ourselves. One sixth former who played a major part in the running of the hostel before he was called up into the navy, was Richard Baker, later to become famous as a broadcaster.

To return to our arrival at Northampton station: a very bleak introduction to a very bleak town. Situated in the middle of England, some locals boasted that it was the most central place in England, but I think that honour belonged to somewhere nearby. The town itself did not lay claim to any special virtue except for its fame as the shoe-making centre of the country. I later came to recognise that the countryside surrounding the town was, in places, quite beautiful, but at a time when cars were a rarity and petrol severely rationed, one did not have an opportunity to appreciate the countryside. The few cars we saw on the road on that first day already had blackout hoods on the headlamps, and as they were nearly all black in colour (in deference to Henry Ford), the bleakness of the place was intensified. For some reason I noted that all the cars had the same letters on their number plates (previously in London there were so many variations that they became anonymous). They displayed either the letter "VV" or "ARP". This last was of interest since it also stood for "Air Raid Precautions", and the civilian population that had been enlisted to protect us in the event of a bombing attack, walked around with the letters "ARP" prominent on their helmets. For many years afterwards, any car I saw with either of these combinations of letters was looked upon with affectionate nostalgia.

The depiction of evacuees carrying a case for temporary clothing and a bag of provisions, including tins of spam, evaporated milk and condensed milk, digestive biscuits and a bar of chocolate, is quite correct, as were the labels on our coats with our name and identification written on it. We were lined up in the now familiar crocodile line and marched off from the station along the road leading from what the Americans call "downtown", up to the more affluent area of town, stopping every now and again at a house where the man or woman in charge (known as the billeting officer) would knock or ring at the front door asking if they could accommodate one or more of us. Because we had originally been left behind and arrived later than the others, many of the promising looking houses had already accepted their quota of "the kids from London" and we became used to seeing a polite but regretful negative nod of the head from the occupants. My brother and I found ourselves at the front of the line (or more accurately, followed our nature which was to stay with us through life, of wanting to be the first in everything we did!), and accordingly at one of the first houses still available the lady came out, looked along the line, and said she would "take the two boys at the front". Accordingly we were the first to be billeted and were not aware of how far the others had to walk before being found a home. My sister was taken in with another girl to a house round the corner that turned out to belong to the brother of the gentleman that accepted us. The family were quite charming, consisting of husband, wife and two grown up daughters, named Madge and

Betty. He was sub (or assistant) editor of the local paper, and they treated us very kindly, if perhaps at a distance. We managed to stay with them a whole year before they found the strain too much and asked if we could go elsewhere. For the next few months we were lodged in a boarding house, while a home was found for us. My abiding memories of the boarding house are of the elderly, austere landlady who treated us as lodgers rather than two young boys in need of a home, and the one other long-stay boarder who was a middle-aged commercial traveller. He was a man of few words where we were concerned, but had the irritating habit of chewing every mouthful of food a total of 32 times before allowing it to start on its long digestive journey through his alimentary canal. After a time, one could not help but be riveted to his mouth, counting the number of chews in case he missed one or allowed himself the luxury of an extra chew.

Our parents were not very happy about their two sons living as lodgers, and set about looking for somewhere else we could live. Having organised an introduction to the local senior billeting officer and expressed their concern, he spoke to a personal friend of his who agreed to "give it a try", and arrangements were made for us to move in.

In the new home we found the family were warm and welcoming and put up with us for as long we wanted to stay. There were two children in the family, a girl the same age as my brother and a boy two years younger than myself. Considering the circumstances, we all got on well together, which is a tribute to not only the parents, but to the younger members as well, who must have had their noses put out of joint to a certain extent, but never let it show.

Recently watching a TV series on evacuation, I was struck by the way the participants tended to look back on it as being a very traumatic time. This was not my experience, and on reflection, I can only judge it as an interesting and sometimes exciting time. Certain factors, I believe, helped me to survive the experience relatively unscathed. First the decision of my parents to keep us together, and our long farm holidays over the previous five summers had accustomed us to the idea of being away from home, while still being part of a family. The fact that we could each continue at our own schools may have been fortuitous but it also ensured the continuity of our education, even though it took place in a different environment. The good nature and generosity of our hosts avoided some of the physical, and even, in some cases, cruel influences that having to live with resentful strangers must have created. Being only sixty miles from London meant that our parents could visit us from time to time, avoiding any feeling of being abandoned that was present in many cases. In addition the rather odd but very real psychological mechanism that exerts itself in stressful circumstances came into play. I refer to the feelings of: "however dangerous the situation is – nothing unpleasant is going to happen to me or those close to me". This feeling was reinforced by the relative absence of serious disasters occurring to our immediate family. As I write this, I realise that I have also succumbed to the psychological mechanism of denial: in fact, my sister's fiancé was a prisoner of war in Germany for four years, having been captured after the surrender in Crete. His brother, a paratroops officer, was killed in action in Italy. My other sister's brother-in-law was a prisoner of war of the Japanese. In addition, our house in Willesden was bombed and made uninhabitable, although fortunately my parents had taken a weekend off in the country to escape the blitz on the night it happened. Finally the bank where my father worked was in the heart of the City, and was destroyed by bombing and consequent fire. Obviously when set against the experiences of some others, it is still possible to say we had a relatively safe war. No known members of my family lived in continental Europe, so the ghastly experiences of those with the same religion that we had escaped us.

The term "phoney war" has a special significance for me as exemplified by some of the episodes I experienced. It is only with hindsight that I realise it was quite a dangerous time, but as I have already said, the main feeling at the time was one of excitement rather than fear. I remember clearly my first air raid. The war was only a few days old and although Northampton could boast only one bomb (which landed in a graveyard) during the entire war, it did occasionally lie on the flight path of German bombers flying elsewhere (on the night Coventry was so heavily bombed and its Cathedral destroyed, it was quite noisy over Northampton and the flames of the burning buildings could just be seen on the horizon). On the night to which I am referring, an aircraft was spotted making its way towards Northampton and the air raid siren bleated its warning. The house we were living in had built an Anderson shelter in the garden, and all six of us trooped out to the shelter, where we sat for about two hours until the all clear sounded. I was terrified to the point of crying, but oddly, after that experience, which finished so tamely with nothing happening, I never felt fear during an air raid again. Even during the summer of 1941 when we were spending a few days with relations in London and the blitz was at its height, I quite happily lay in bed listening to the alternating booming of bombs and anti-aircraft fire. It was an adventure to go up to town the next morning and walk down Oxford Street observing the smashed windows and debris of the shops. As I walked along the shattered street I picked up pieces of shrapnel to keep as souvenirs, which I kept for many years as a reminder of the times in which we were living.

By the summer of 1942, the war at home had quietened down somewhat, although horrifying things were still going on overseas. We were allowed to stay at home in London over the summer holidays. As our house was uninhabitable, my parents had found a flat in Swiss Cottage, where we lived until well after the war. All four of us children were married from the same block of flats, although after the family reduced in size following my sisters' weddings, we transferred to a smaller flat in the same block. After my mother died in 1977, my father continued living there on his own for a short time before he found the strain too much and moved into a home in Hampstead for his remaining days. During these holidays, my mother decided that she wanted me back home again and as our school had re-opened in Willesden, it was not a problem for me to return to London, although my brother stayed in Northampton for a further year. I did not find it too difficult to make new friends at school, and also there were five or six young boys of my age who lived in the flats, with whom I became friendly. Living in Swiss Cottage and having to travel to Willesden to school created a problem, but I managed to persuade my parents to buy me a bike, much against their will. Not any old bike, but a bright orange, low handlebar, three-gear Claude Butler sport's bike. Actually, it was my mother who I managed to persuade to fork out all of £15 on the bike, and the look on my father's face when confronted with the new purchase was not to be missed. In spite of his pessimistic prophesy that "it was even money chances that I would kill myself on it", I managed to survive the odds and enjoyed many hours showing off my acquisition. For the journey from home to school I had to navigate Swiss Cottage, Kilburn High Road and Willesden High Road. I wonder if either the bike or I would successfully achieve this in the current climate of heavy traffic and bicycle crime! I also remember the occasional excursion, cycling along the North Circular Road as far as Richmond and Kew Gardens – not something I would relish today.

For a year or two it was almost as if the war had ended, but one day in 1944 the sirens sounded just after I had arrived at school and we were all sent to the shelter. Usually this would be for no more than an hour before the all clear sounded and we resumed lessons, but on this occasion there was no all clear. After lunch one of my form mates arrived at the school in great excitement: he informed us breathlessly that he had seen a German plane shot down. He was mistaken: it was our first introduction to the German V1 or "flying bomb". Hitler used these ghastly devices, together with unmanned rockets or V2s, in a last hopeless attempt to avert defeat. Fortunately he failed, but their impact was quite frightening inasmuch as they could land and create severe damage just about anywhere. As with everything else in life, familiarity bred contempt and very soon we found ourselves ignoring the air raid warnings and going about our everyday life. One had to accept that when you went to school in the morning you might not have a home to come back to that evening. The flat we lived in was on the fifth floor and the front looked due south over the centre of London and the back due north. Quite frequently we would hear the drone of the flying bomb and would then see it approaching out of the south-facing window, hear it directly overhead (at which point we would start praying!) and then watch it disappear northwards out of the back window. Eventually the engine sound would cut out and the plane reverted to being a bomb and one might or might not see it hurtling towards the ground, finishing up as a plume of smoke hiding the destruction and death it had caused. When the V2 rockets started, one no longer had the "luxury" of seeing them coming, but only hearing the bang as they exploded (if you heard the bang, then you knew you were all right).

Between 1942 and 1945 I continued living at home and attending school. Attendance at the Youth Hostel in Northampton had now been changed to attending the local youth club, where more new friends were made. Table tennis and amateur dramatics filled up a lot of the time, and I began to take a greater interest in the opposite sex. On one occasion, I remember, I was sitting watching enviously as some of the others danced to a smooth American band (probably Glen Miller), when a young lady came up to me and said, "You are fourteen years old now, it is time to learn to dance." It was great fun learning, but judging by my future experiences, it was not wholly successful and my dancing skills still tend to rely on my using the waltz or quickstep movements no matter what rhythm the band is playing.

I was now approaching the age of sixteen and although not eligible for call up to the services, might have been able to join the ARP, although in what capacity is unclear. As it turned out, my sole contribution was to do occasional fire watching, and I became expert at using the stirrup pump to douse any fires that might be started by incendiary bombs (although I was never called upon to use the pump in anger!). In June 1945 I sat what was then called "school certificate" or "matric". This was just one month after victory in the war against Germany had been achieved, so-called VE Day. The celebrations, mainly in the streets, are still vivid in my memory. I had taken the tube to the West End and had been given licence, for one day at least, to talk to anyone and to hug and kiss any girl to whom I was attracted. At the age of sixteen this was indeed a privilege. I met some other young people from the club, and we all went to one of the boys' flat in Baker Street. The only down side to the whole day was having to walk back home after midnight having drunk rather too much, but on the whole the euphoria of the day overcame the depression. Final victory over the Japanese (VJ Day) came about three months later in August 1945. The whole process of celebration was repeated, but although historically it was a more important day, at the time, trying to reproduce the euphoria of three months previously was difficult to achieve.

If asked now if I had a good war, I would have to answer that for the most part it was not too bad (speaking purely of my own experiences). In retrospect and from the viewpoint of adulthood, I would not be able to give such an optimistic reply. The realisation of how close we came to disaster, and what would have been the inevitable outcome for us if Germany, under Hitler, would have been the victors, does not bear thinking about – and perhaps that is why, at the time, we did not think about it. I often ask myself what action I might have taken pre-1939 if I had been an adult with my family as they are now, and living in Germany. With hindsight there is no doubt that the wiser members of the Jewish community packed their belongings and left between 1933 and 1939, but had I been a successful practising doctor, with many friends of all religions among my acquaintances, would I have felt secure enough to stay? I am sure I would have found it very difficult to leave. Others, of course, were not so fortunate and had a lousy war: they were truly terrible times, but I was fortunate in so many ways, and my life was not changed by my experiences. For all its faults, those of us born and brought up in Britain are very lucky indeed.

CHAPTER IV

Becoming a Doctor

The question, "Why did you become a doctor?" is one frequently asked. The stock answer usually given is, "because I want to benefit mankind, and doctoring is a good way of achieving this" (to say nothing of the security and good living it gives one!). An American comedian, whose name I do not remember – it was of the era of Bob Hope, Jack Benny, George Burns et al (those were the days!) – put it rather more crudely by stating that "he could not think of any other occupation that allowed you to undress the wife of your best friend and be paid for the privilege". I can't speak for American doctors, but I genuinely do not believe that this is a motivation for the vast majority of the profession, even though anyone watching some of the TV medical horror shows may be tempted to believe it is so. After much reflection, I believe my own motivation was curiosity. I am very interested in what makes the human race function, why we behave as we do and why we react so differently to similar situations. As a doctor one is given "carte blanche" to ask all these questions, and although it takes many years of experience to interpret what one is being told, I believe the years spent satisfyingly in a medical career has answered many of the questions about which I have previously only conjectured. Some years ago, I gave this answer to an American physician I had met casually and incongruously at a show in a Las Vegas casino. It was met with complete disbelief, but it did not take very long to recognise he was in denial (who knows, maybe the wife of his best friend . . . ?)

My first memory of wanting to become a doctor is still very clear. I was eleven years old, and a school friend showed me a leather pouch he treasured. Inside was a dissecting set of scalpels and forceps. Heaven knows from where he got them, but I thought the forceps were great and if I became a doctor, I too could possess such wonderful items (it is lucky my fantasy was for the forceps and not the scalpels otherwise I might have finished up as a hoodie and added to the appalling statistics of knife crime on the streets). From that day on, I never contemplated any other career than medicine. I did not find studying in my school years too difficult, but to me playing cricket was equally as important as studying. I overcame the dilemma by getting up during the summer months at 5am in the morning and doing two hours studying so I could play cricket in the evening. Funnily enough I have tried passing on the same advice to my grandsons, but there have been no takers.

My alma mater was The London Hospital, at the time one of the great teaching institutions. Teaching was by lecture and observation in the wards and in outpatients. Some of the Consultants were also great teachers, attracting students (undergraduate and postgraduate) from all over the world. We hung upon their every word, greatly influenced by the way they projected their personalities and (unfortunately) didactic views. It took some years in practice before I realised that sometimes the best teachers were also the most dangerous. Their overbearing views, put across with such apparent sincerity, left us practising a form of medicine that showed no evidence of advancing or of taking the views of the patients into account. At one lecture on neurology, a distinguished physician with a great reputation for teaching, started a lecture to a number of GPs hoping to increase their knowledge and aptitude, with the words: "Gentlemen and ladies, I bring you great comfort. Every GP I have come across is worried that the headache about which a patient complains in a busy surgery is the first sign of a brain tumour, and he will miss it. Do not worry. Only less than one in a hundred will actually be due to a tumour, and all the others will be benign." Exactly! It is that single one that gives us the nightmare, since in medicine, unlike the law, you cannot base a diagnosis on the balance of probabilities. Put another way, a friend once told me that his father had said to him that if you were one of a hundred people held hostage and informed that one of you would be shot the following morning, the odds of it being you is only 100:1, but all of you would no doubt have a sleepless night.

Perhaps it has gone too far the other way today, with doctors scared to give an opinion for fear of being contradicted or sued. Algorithms and evidence-based medicine have added to the problem by taking away the "art" of medicine and replacing it with complete uniformity. I used to call this "chocolate machine medicine": you put sixpence in the machine and a bar of chocolate is immediately produced. Michael Balint (about whom I have written elsewhere) opened our eyes to the concept of the "overall diagnosis" (in general practice anyway). Instead of the "traditional diagnosis" usually expressed in one or two words and which could be found in "International Classification of Diseases" and even given a number to identify it, the diagnosis should be expressed in physical, psychological and social terms. He called the former the traditional diagnosis and the latter the overall diagnosis. The idea has been partially embraced within general practice, but is too often, I fear, achieved only in the breach and not the actuality.

Before leaving the subject, let me recount a memory of one of the great teachers I was privileged to come across. A. E. Clarke Kennedy (I never did discover what the "A E" stood for) was dean of the medical college as well as a general physician, a breed not only rare but driven to extinction by hyper-specialisation today. He was a tall, lean figure and his ward rounds would often equate the differential diagnosis of the patient being discussed with horse race betting. He would ask us all in turn for a possible diagnosis, and then ask, "and if this was a horse race what are the odds of your diagnosis being correct?" In this way we would work through from favourite to 100 to 1 outsider. He would then remind us that in making a diagnosis, the favourite was likely to win, but outsiders did sometimes come first past the post. What a lesson! What an influence it had on me! I have still not lost my interest in gambling on the horses! Later I realised that the adages, "common things occur more commonly" or even, "if you see a bird in your garden it is more likely to be a sparrow than a vulture", although more succinct, were equally true.

Without wishing to fall into the trap of "those were the days", there is one aspect of teaching medicine that has changed greatly, and not, in my opinion, for the better. One of the benefits of studying medicine in the British system was in the way it was a combination of lecturing, home studying and, arguably the most effective method, learning by the bedside – a form of apprentice-ship to which we all submitted for the final three years of our undergraduate degree. Sitting by the bedside discussing the illness with the patient helped us understand the sociological aspect. Watching how they reacted to the circumstances of their illness helped understand the psychological side. Assisting at surgical operations and in outpatients guided us towards the practical side of medicine. Attending the post mortem room to see the process of disease that had stricken the patient we had clerked gave an insight into the meaning of the word "disease". We were scornful of the students from some other countries whose complete knowledge of medicine was based on lecture and demonstration. They may have known the textbooks by heart but I firmly believe that we understood the subject more fully. Unfortunately, time has seen the financial aspects of practising medicine overtake the caring side with consequent lessening of the time allowed to study the patient before the next "customer" is admitted. Slowly, but surely, we are deluding ourselves that much of the learning we did was a waste of time. "Faking it" programmes on TV have led to the conclusion that "with an intensive short course, anyone can do anything". How convenient that a shorter course can be justified by maintaining that more extensive bookwork can outweigh the hands-on approach. Money is saved; more people can become doctors and help the shortage that is universal; a fairer distribution of medical students will be allowed into medical school, and worst of all, "centres of excellence" – implying unequal quality of care – will be abolished and all hospitals will be judged the same, namely second-class.

CHAPTER V

Early Influences and Experiences

I entered medical school in 1947, a day I still remember as if it was only a few years ago rather than over 60 years. I often reflect on the idea that if I go back from the time I became a medical student, as many years as I have been qualified, I would arrive at the year 1886, 10 years before my own father was born, and the heyday of Queen Victoria's reign. Only six years after the death of Anthony Trollope, the great Victorian novelist, whose works I have read almost in their entirety (and many twice or thrice over), and a time when medical science was still quite primitive in contrast to our present knowledge.

I left medical school, on qualification, in 1952, and the period 1947 to 1952 was significant in several respects. First, from 1945 only 10% of students could be accepted straight from school at the age of 18 or thereabouts. The rest were made up of men and women who had served in the armed services (or equivalent war duty). All these would have had between one and six years war experience: many were married with families of their own and their first priority was to "get on with it" and qualify as soon as possible. They had little time to enjoy the excesses usually attributed to student life, and although they spoke very little of their wartime experience, they included among their number many who had outstanding war careers with medals for bravery to show for it, and some with heartrending experiences or years wasted as prisoners of war of the Germans or the Japanese. Others had a "lucky war" and I remember one in particular who qualified as a fighter pilot in 1940 (the year of the Battle of Britain), but went through the remaining four years without once having to go into combat. At each posting, by the time he arrived the war had passed on to another field of combat. The effect these mature students had on those of us who were fresh-faced rookies from school, was that we had to grow up quickly to compete with them, as a result of which our student behaviour was rather more sober than the impression one gets from reading or seeing books and films such as *Doctor in the House*.

In addition, 1947 was the first year in which it was compulsory for medical schools to accept at least 10% women (or in the case of the all-female Royal Free Hospital, 10% men). This certainly made our time at college more sociable – and we also learnt more of the social skills that women demanded of men: women were still yearning after equality, but had not yet reached it. Finally, 1952, the year I qualified, was the last year in which you could become fully registered as a medical practitioner as soon as you had passed your final qualifying exam. After 1952 it was obligatory to spend at least one year provisionally registered before you could consider entering general practice. Later still, it became obligatory to spend a minimum of three years vocational training after one year's provisional registration (spent as a house officer in hospital). Compulsory membership of The Royal College of General Practitioners has still to be enforced though it is on the cards. In effect this means that contemporary GPs have had four years extra training over the minimum requirement when I qualified. I have no doubt this is beneficial to both the profession and patients, but in my own case it meant that a lot of my early preparation for general practice was self taught and although I believe it worked in my case, many young doctors fell by the wayside and it led to an under-trained branch of the medical profession who had to compete for resources and prestige against other highly trained specialties. It also meant that anyone whose father, or other close family member or friend, was a GP, could join them as a fully fledged GP the day after they qualified (assuming they had reason to avoid National Service, a minimum of two years in the armed forces, which was compulsory at that time). Avoiding National Service for some was not too difficult, the trick being to have a medical condition severe enough to avoid onerous service duties, but not bad enough to be life or comfort threatening. In one famous case, a recruit avoided military service because of a condition known as "hallux rigidus" (a fixed and stiff big toe joint), but later was fit enough to play cricket at test match level. It was, perhaps, more difficult to achieve for doctors, as they entered the Services under the best possible condition: immediate officer status, non-combatant and serving in one's chosen profession. "Square bashing" training was set at a minimum; in my case one afternoon set aside during the first month's indoctrination training to be an officer. Even this was rained off! For my part, I joined the RAF and volunteered to increase the compulsory two years to three as this gave me 'short service commission' status with extra pay and advantaged living accommodation – important to me as I was newly married with a recently born child. I do not resent a moment of my time in the RAF; it was very rewarding.

Having passed my final exams, I was certain that I was fully able to act as adviser, confidant, diagnostician and "all things to all patients", which was the requirement for a competent general practitioner. I believe this was a confidence shared with most of my contemporaries, but many years were to pass and episodes experienced before I realised that this state of nirvana is probably never reached, and those that believe it is, show a lamentable lack of insight. In describing some of the experiences from my early years as a GP I will try and be as truthful as memory will allow, within the bounds of a certain poetic licence; names and identities will obviously be changed for reasons of confidentiality.

Two episodes opened my eyes to the fact that we are very often judged, not on how or why we do things, but only on the obvious outcomes of what we do. The first occurred during my six months as a house surgeon on an Orthopaedic firm whose four consultants included two knights of the realm and one former Scottish rugby international who had a growing reputation as an innovator of new orthopaedic techniques, hitherto thought to be impossible (though nowadays considered routine). One technique he had mastered was to permanently straighten the backs of elderly men bent over double with their head facing the ground, a consequence of untreated *ankylosing spondylitis* of the spine. His technique was to break the spine about one third of the way down from the neck, then reset it and wait for it to knit together, a period of about two to three months during which the patient was completely immobilised within a plaster cast from the neck down. When successful it worked well and left a highly satisfied patient. However, as with so many pioneers and innovators, initial success too often led to over eagerness and small things, like unsuitability in some patients, were conveniently forgotten in the enthusiasm to display and teach one's skills to colleagues equally eager to improve their ability to cure. I had responsibility for the post-operative care of "Arthur", an old man in his seventies, who as well as his crippled and bent back, had type 1 diabetes that was not too well controlled. Being unable to move, and for the first week or so after the operation, unable to eat and drink in the ordered way that is essential for diabetics, he quickly became dehydrated and acidotic (two serious complications of diabetes). It was my job to keep him hydrated and this could only be done by means of an intravenous drip, but unfortunately all his veins were collapsed, which meant having to cut down on them. I had no experience of this technique and due to my inexperience and probable clumsiness I could not succeed in getting the drip that he so desperately needed into a vein or to prevent it coming out. As a result I spent all night being recalled by the nurse on night duty, because the drip was not working or had come out yet again. No doubt the reader will understand my sense of uselessness and frustration, but to my surprise, the next morning I was the toast of all the other patients in the ward, in whose eyes this young doctor had spent all night fighting for a man's life. They had no idea it was my incompetence that had really kept me awake. I did not feel any better, when the registrar the next morning, after a good night's sleep, slipped the drip in and kept it going, with no trouble at all.

The next example, showing the other side of the coin, occurred while I was in the Air Force, stationed in Malta. I was medical officer on duty at Luqa airport (at that time shared between the Maltese Civil Aviation Authority and the RAF), when the alarm bell rang. I was informed that a single passenger fighter aircraft, being ferried to one of the Middle East countries via Malta for refuelling, had crashed on the runway and the pilot was badly injured. I arrived at the scene of the crash at the same time as the ambulance, to find a badly damaged aircraft (which was not my business) and a very severely wounded, barely alive pilot (which was). There was little I could do apart from supervising his transfer into the ambulance and ordering it to take him to the Naval Hospital, which I considered the most appropriately equipped hospital. I firmly believed that the correct behaviour of a doctor in these circumstances was to stay with the patient until responsibility could be passed over to a competent authority: hadn't Hippocrates taught us to cure occasionally, diagnose sometimes and comfort always – or something to that effect? Accordingly I stayed with the pilot until he got to hospital and then made my own way back to the airport. Unfortunately, the pilot did not survive his injuries, but I was very surprised when, instead of being complimented on my actions and humane response to the situation, I was hauled over the coals on two counts. First, a message from the naval bureaucracy informed me that I had no right to take the pilot to their hospital as he was not a serving member of any armed force (country was not important), but a civilian pilot who should have been taken to the local hospital. Although Maltese medical services have always been very good, at that time I do not believe they had the facilities to provide as good a standard of care that was available at the Naval Hospital. Of more serious consequence for me was being called before the commanding officer, to be reprimanded for leaving my place of duty, and therefore the airport, without medical cover for the 90 minutes it had taken me to look after the tragic airman.

I was reminded of this early part of my career recently, when I was on a cruise between Hong Kong and Singapore via the Philippines, Malaysia and Brunei. The cruise was a success; as well as visiting new places, we also met several interesting and multinational fellow guests. One of the places we visited was a small town – more a village really. Not a place, I imagine, that would be familiar to many people, but it was one of the places that suffered very badly during the war against Japan. It was from here that the "death march" started during which, we were told, in the region of 17,000 took part and only a handful survived. The weather on that day was very wet and as a result my wife decided that she would rather stay on board the ship, and I went on my own. About fifteen other intrepid travellers were on the excursion and our first stop was the Christian Church in the town: being a Muslim country, this was considered to be a tourist attraction.

It was a small and not very imposing building, but on entering we were informed that the stained glass window at the back of the church was a gift from Britain to recognise and remember the events of the war. Most visitors did not bother to retreat to the back of the church to view the window more closely, but a few of us did, and my interest in the window was overshadowed by a series of commemorative plaques representing individuals or regiments on display on the wall by the window. My eyes alighted on a plaque portraying the Royal Army Medical Corp (RAMC), but it was in memory of a single individual. Overcome with curiosity I read the inscription in full. It started "In memory of Captain ____ ". Presumably it was in memory of a young doctor who had died while serving his country. It was with increasing horror I noted that the inscription did not continue with the more usual "died in action", or "killed in action" or even "one of the fallen", but merely stated in stark and horrific reality: "Executed on the 7th August 1945." The date was of historical significance, being the day after the first atom bomb was dropped on Hiroshima, but for me it had an added significance. On that day I had passed the first academic hurdle on my way to becoming a doctor, and was about to start my medical training proper. It was also a date on which the end of the war was very much in sight. And by no means of least significance to me, it was the day I first met my wife, and our lives have been intertwined ever since.

I found myself overcome with emotion as these facts sank home: Captain _____ was probably only ten or so years older than me. Instead of looking forward to a career in medicine as I was, his was cruelly cut short while still on the threshold. And that word, "executed", presumably beheaded by the Japanese for a "crime" for which he had no responsibility. The psychological mechanism of identification overcame me, and when I returned to the bus for the next part of the tour, I found myself alone and weeping openly. Alone, as he must have been in his last, dark days.

CHAPTER VI

Teaching and Learning

Teaching comes in many forms including lecturing, apprenticeship, self-experience and seminar discussions. Learning should be a consequence of teaching, but if one relies on lecturing alone, as so many of us tend to do, one is left at the mercy of the lecturer and his personal knowledge and biases. Perhaps the most dangerous of the species are lecturers with biased or even incorrect views, but whose expertise at lecturing is outstanding. Fortunately those with these attributes are more likely to go into politics than teaching. Over the years I have come across lecturers who have been so good at imparting their message, that it has taken many years of personal experience to realise that the knowledge to which I had been exposed, or even been influenced by, was incorrect and possibly dangerous. I think I agree largely with Miss Jean Brodie's view on education. She said, "to me education is a leading out of what is already there in the pupil's soul. [To Miss Mackay] it is a putting in of something that is not there, and that is not what I call education, I call it intrusion."

My Chemistry master at school was a truly didactic teacher. He recounted how he, himself, as a schoolboy had been taught by a master whose method was to take hold of an unfortunate pupil and repeat the mantra, with a hit over alternate ears with each word: "Base (hit right ear) plus (hit left ear) acid (hit right ear) equals (hit left ear) salt (hit right ear) plus (hit left ear) water." In the natural order of things, a rather useless piece of information – but a formula I have never forgotten even though I do not recommend the method used. From medical school, I can still hear with joy the dulcet Dublin accent (that soft Irish accent so far removed from the coarser accent of Northern Ireland) of our anatomy teacher, Professor Boyd, whose delivery of the dry facts of anatomy made the subject come to life as we sat in thrall of his oratory. He was the co-author of a textbook of anatomy (Hamilton Boyd and Mossman), but reading it came nowhere near the experience of hearing him. I must admit I do not remember very much of the contents of the lectures; but in my mind I can still *hear* him.

When analysing the attendance at a lecture, it is important to differentiate between hearing and listening. Hearing is the physiological act of the ears accepting sound. Listening is the act of understanding, interpreting and appraising what one has heard. Hearing without listening can lead only to ignorance or lack of judgment. My experience in general practice has confirmed the importance of this distinction, and listening to the patient, rather than merely hearing what they say, is the difference between the good and merely average GP. The years I spent working with Balint Groups opened my eyes to this phenomenon. Michael Balint was a psychoanalyst who ran seminar groups of GPs who learned, through shared experiences and discussions, the importance of the doctor patient relationship in reaching a greater understanding of the patient's needs, many of which were not openly expressed or even not consciously recognised by the patient. Under his influence, and that of his wife, Enid Balint, also a psychoanalyst working at the Tavistock Clinic, I came to understand that within a consultation, it is as if there is an old fashioned wireless in the room that is switched off. Surrounding it are radio waves, but these remain unrecognised and unheard until the wireless is switched on, at which point it recognises their presence. However, before distinguishing the non-recognisable cackle that one then hears, the instrument has to be tuned into a station. If the station is the wrong one, the direction in which the consultation proceeds can be completely wrong and irrelevant to the patient's needs. If the correct station has been chosen (and finding this is the true art of medicine), further exploration can be achieved by using the fine tuner, and at this point, if it can be reached, the consultation can be judged to be successful. If a specific disease is involved, the importance of evidence-based medicine is a factor, but if the problem lies within the psyche rather than the soma, interpretation is of greater importance. Unfortunately, this principle is being increasingly ignored, and the distorted conclusion has been reached that "where there is no evidence there is no disease". This can be likened to the theoretical argument that asks the question "if a tree falls down in a forest in which there is no one present to hear it, has a sound actually been created?" In other words, if a patient complains, but no evidence for disease can be found, is there a disease actually present? Recognition of the principles taught by Balint and his followers are in danger of being forgotten in a system that gives financial rewards to those who can produce number crunching evidence but none to those who continue to give prominence to the art of medicine.

A fellow GP from my past, and one who had the gift of imparting knowledge in a way that was highly influential (to me, anyway), was Marshall Marinker. He was responsible for opening my eyes to a better understanding of what is meant when we are unwell. I think I may have adapted his views to be more in keeping with my own and if I have I apologise, but it is worth repeating. We are all aware of what we mean by the word *health*, but there is no satisfactory word for the opposite, and he coined the word *unhealth*. Though not a true word, its meaning is clear. So-called *unhealth* can be divided into three categories for which words that are normally used interchangeably can be used. I refer to *illness*, *disease* and *sickness*. For greater understanding of the processes through which a patient travels when consulting a doctor, these words can be given more specific meanings:

1) *Illness*. This is what the patient feels when consulting the doctor. "I have a pain, Doctor." Or: "I feel ill."
2) *Disease*. This is the diagnosis the doctor makes of the illness (either correctly or incorrectly) after the appropriate history taking, examination and investigations. This diagnosis then becomes the patient's property – and heaven help another

doctor who tries to alter it! (How often does a consultation commence "It's *my* migraine", or "It's *my* blood pressure"?) Changing the diagnosis may not only be difficult but might be impossible: for instance if Doctor A has diagnosed migraine, Doctor B is likely to have great difficulty in convincing the patient that it may be a tension headache. However, there is a hierarchy of disease that may influence the outcome: if Doctor C says it may be a brain tumour, this diagnosis is likely to outbid migraine in the mind of the patient.

3) *Sickness*. This describes the state one is allowed to enter if the doctor has diagnosed a disease. Where this is the case, the patient is entitled to take to his "sick bed", take "sick leave", or have a "sick note" to stay away from work. He or she is also entitled to the full sympathy of family and friends, and it implies that the diagnosis is a genuine illness, and not just in the mind.

The inference to be taken from this classification is that if the patient attends the doctor feeling ill, and the doctor diagnoses a disease there is no problem in entering the sick role and receiving the secondary benefits that this incurs. The problem arises when the doctor fails to find anything specifically wrong to which he can give a named diagnosis, a situation well recognised in general practice. This is a common cause of disagreement that may develop between the patient and the doctor, creating a barrier to true understanding. As a consequence the doctor may be tempted to give a name to an illness rather too quickly and before it can be confirmed; in this way he enters a comfort zone, but the outcome for the patient may not be helpful. It is, perhaps, the reason for the frequently expressed criticism that doctors are too often incorrect, their diagnoses too often proving wrong.

The present fashion tends towards what I call chocolate-machine medicine, whereby you put your coin in to a vending machine (the symptoms), and out comes a bar of chocolate (the diagnosis). This system has encouraged the loss of the art of medicine, replaced by something that, with the help of an algorithm, anyone can practice as long as they have undergone a few weeks' tuition. Judge for yourself which is more likely to improve patient care and management.

I have always had an interest in teaching and it was fortunate that during the years I was in practice, teaching of general practice became fashionable: previously all teaching of medicine was felt to be the prerogative of hospital consultants, and GPs were merely expected to sit at their feet soaking up their pearls of wisdom, which were mainly relevant to hospital medicine and too often bore little reference to what was actually experienced in general practice. I remember attending a refresher course for GPs run by the local hospital consultants. The front two rows were, as usual, occupied by those whom I privately thought of as The Scribes. They would sit with their notepads and pens at the ready, copying down every word that was uttered by the god-like figure before them. I actually witnessed one elderly doctor faithfully reproducing the words: "For a headache give two aspirin."

In the 1950s, under the influence of the recently formed College of General Practitioners (later to be given the Royal Charter), it was becoming recognised that the responsibility for the teaching of actual GP practice fell onto the shoulders of GPs themselves. The opportunity arose for us to teach, and many of us seized it enthusiastically. Unlike some of our hospital colleagues, we realised that, alone, having a medical qualification and experience of practice was not enough to make us successful teachers. We needed to learn about teaching itself. A group of about 14 of us formed the London Teachers' Workshop, and met fortnightly at a lovely house overlooking Primrose Hill that belonged to John Horder. This was noble of him since, having offered his house for our meetings, he then discovered they were held on days when he was unavailable: very much our loss, since his output would have been most helpful. I first came across John as a student, when the Medical College at The London Hospital started a scheme of appointing tutors to groups of students. I was allocated to him and ever since I have looked upon him with the greatest of respect. Although not officially a mentor, I am sure he would have accepted the role if I had ever requested it. Sadly he died in 2012. His wisdom, humanity and many other gifts will be long remembered.

At our meetings, we discussed topics related to teaching rather in the same way that Balint seminars were held. In fact a fair proportion of us were also followers of Balint. We were also fortunate in securing the guidance of Professor Furneaux, an educationalist. He rarely attended the meetings in person, but notes of our discussions were sent to him and he wrote back with any advice he thought appropriate. One very important outcome resulted. At one of our meetings he explained that teachers were beginning a new form of training in which they role-played situations and then discussed them at length. They were finding it very helpful and he suggested we should try it as a means of increasing our expertise in teaching. The suggestion was greeted with enthusiasm, and we arranged to go away to Jordans, a Quaker Retreat in Buckinghamshire, for a weekend, to practice role-play on ourselves to see if it might be a helpful additional tool in medical training. I believe Professor Knox, who had been one of the first professors of general practice to be appointed, was already using the method with his students, but he was not, unfortunately, a member of our workshop. The rest, as they say, is history. This form of teaching has become almost standard. Most students find it helpful, but some find it difficult to act out the role of a patient. A later development of role-play (and I am not certain whether it is more beneficial or not) has seen professional actors employed as patients. Although they have proved to be very successful in this, it has taken away one advantage that playing the patient has for the medical student or doctor: namely to gain an increased insight into the feelings of the patient. During our weekend away, I had played the part of a patient in which I had made use of a consultation that had occurred during the previous week and about which I was feeling uncomfortable. This concerned a patient who had demanded, rather than requested, a certificate of sickness for a reason that I found difficult to justify.

A member of his family was ill and he needed time off, and while I was sympathetic to his need, I did not necessarily believe this was the correct way to solve the problem. (I think in later years I became more sympathetic to this type of demand; or perhaps just more compliant!) I was aware that this particular patient was having a problem with his wife, who was threatening to leave him. However, this was not the reason he was requesting a certificate. So I commenced the role-play consultation by aggressively telling the doctor I needed a certificate for my workplace because I was not feeling well and my boss was demanding to see a doctor's certificate. Not surprisingly, the role-playing doctor asked what exactly was wrong with me that made me unfit for work. I grew progressively more difficult, refusing to give any more details but merely reiterating that all I wanted was a certificate. As the atmosphere of the consultation became fierier, our voices began to rise to a crescendo as we squared up to each other. I remember that at this point I specifically thought to myself (as the patient), "If only he would ask me about the problem with my wife. Then I'll be nice to him." I think it was probably the first time I really entered the role of being a patient and recognising what the patient feels, rather than focusing on the doctor's needs to make a diagnosis. As our experimental workshop progressed we came to recognise that in role-play the doctor actually feels what emotions a patient undergoes during what, to the doctor, is a routine consultation. I believe that my experience is far from unique and role-play has become a positive force in teaching skills, complementary to merely diagnosing, prescribing, imparting bad news and management.

In a recent conversation with another member of the workshop, I was reminded that I was the first doctor at the retreat to volunteer to act the patient. As such I became the first person to use role-play as a teaching tool in general practice. A very small footprint in the course of medical history perhaps, but one that makes me very proud nonetheless.

CHAPTER VII

Myths and Misses

Over the years many so-called medical facts have become established in the folklore of the profession. Experience has taught me that many of them need to be questioned and very often do not hold up to scrutiny. It is about some of these, which I call "myths", that I wish to write about. "Misses" does not, as it might appear, refer to married ladies, but to episodes that nearly happened to me but did not materialise.

Many doctors, if asked, will assert "all patients are the same when I treat them, and I do not favour one above another". But is this really true? Certainly at the time of treating someone, their background, ethnicity, character or anything else that distinguishes them from their fellows, does not affect the degree of care they receive. Presumably, even if Hitler were to collapse in front of you with a heart attack, one's medical instincts would overcome the personal hatred one might well feel. But I came to question this myth in everyday practice, after reading a book by Eric Byrne, a psychiatrist, who wrote *Games People Play* in the early 1960s. It received a lot of newspaper coverage, as a result of which it became a bestseller. Although reaching a large readership, it was, in fact, quite a learned textbook and I suspect misunderstood, or not understood at all, by many of its readers and the book probably spent more time on the bookshelf than actually being read. The "games" of the title referred more to the meaning of the word used by Stephen Potter in his satirical look at "gamesmanship": how an individual can beat an opponent in any walk of life by shifting the rules of play, if necessary by cheating, in order to gain an unfair advantage. The behaviour of some of the players on the championship tennis circuit during the era of John

McEnroe will give some idea of what is meant. Byrne theorised that within a doctor/patient relationship, there was a "game", usually at an unconscious level, in which the two sides vied for superiority. He also postulated that in real life situations people interacted by giving a series of what he called "strokes" to each other. For example if one meets an acquaintance in the street, it is customary to ask, "How are you?" One does not expect a medical history as the response; normally the reply will be, "Fine thank you." (Recently I rang an old friend who I had not been in contact with for a couple of years, and made the usual polite enquiry of asking him how he was. He replied that he was quite well, but if my enquiry was a genuine request for information it would take about forty minutes to give me a complete update on his health.) At this point, the first enquirer will expect to be asked back, "And how are you?" If this response is not forthcoming, he will feel very put out and resentful, but if it is he will feel a sense of gratification. By the same token, when a doctor treats a patient, he will only feel fully rewarded for his efforts if there is some return for his investment. This is what might be defined as "job satisfaction".

What then does the doctor expect from a patient that will give him the gratification he is seeking? Or alternatively, what makes him feel frustrated and angry if he does not receive it? The least one expects, is to be thanked for one's trouble. This can be best illustrated by the anger felt by the doctor when told by the patient that he is entitled to demand the doctor's attention because "he pays his stamp" and that's the doctor's job. This may be an irrational feeling, but very real nonetheless. Gratitude from a patient is a difficult gift to refuse, but if it leads to permanent dependence on the doctor, it is not very healthy. Satisfaction may also be experienced if the patient proves to be emotionally and/or intellectually compatible with the doctor. A variation of this is if the patient is a person of interest, especially if well known or famous. (You don't agree? Then why do politicians always get privileged treatment when they are unwell, thus allowing them to extol the wonders of their experiences of the National Health

Service, which very often are by no means the same as experienced by the "ordinary man on the Clapham bus"?) Then there is the patient who presents with an illness that the doctor is capable of diagnosing and, even better, treating successfully. Very few medical experiences are more frustrating than when the doctor finds nothing wrong (in the "traditional diagnosis" sense of the word). Then, if the patient persists in his search for a cause, he may become the victim of the doctor's anger and is made the scapegoat for daring to feel ill. Allied to this is the hierarchy of diagnosis. A patient with a serious or rare disease is much more likely to be treated with consideration than one with a "common or garden" disorder. Being able to say, "I am a cancer sufferer" has become almost a badge of honour, deserving extra sympathy and consideration. Although it may have pejorative overtones, the payment of a fee by the patient or the presentation of a gift, is likely to produce some feeling of gratification in the doctor. Patients may treat the private doctor with more respect than one practising within the NHS, which in turn is gratifying to the ego of the doctor. Finally, and this in my opinion is the greatest gift of all that can be bestowed, is for the patient to get better. One has to add the caveat that "but only if the patient recognises the role the doctor has played in the success of his treatment". There is nothing more disconcerting than the patient who returns after a successful consultation (in the judgment of the doctor), who first gives you a glow of pleasure by informing you that they feel much better, but only to dispel this by adding, "I had to stop your medicine as it made me feel so ill, but decided to pull myself together and this did the trick". (Or the variation, "but the osteopath/acupuncturist/another doctor down the road soon got to the bottom of it and put me right".)

"The post-mortem room is claimed to be the 'Palace of Truth'". This was instilled into us at medical school, both by the senior clinicians and pathologists. I remember attending many "clinical/pathological conferences" in which a very complicated case would be presented and discussed by all the disciplines present, and then finally the pathologist would reveal the true diagnosis as found at post mortem (the patient involved in the case always being dead!). As comforting as belief in this is, it is not always true, as illustrated by the following experience I had while working as a trainee in Paddington in 1956. Let us call her Annabel, as I have long forgotten her name. She was a young West Indian lady, about 29 years of age. She consulted me with what appeared to be a cold and I advised her to take aspirin and gargle. I was shocked about three days later when I received a call from the coroner's officer to say that she had been found dead in her bed: no obvious reason had been found but a friend had remembered that she had visited the doctor a few days earlier. Could I, he asked, throw any light on the puzzle? Not surprisingly my first reaction was one of guilt and despair at having apparently missed some serious illness, which had proved fatal. I was informed that a post mortem examination would be necessary, and in view of my interest and feelings of guilt, I requested permission to be present, which was granted (it was a lot easier in those days to follow up one's cases). To this day I remember the pathologist, who happened to be one of the leaders in the profession and famous in many cases of murder in which he had been involved as an expert, saying that the only abnormal signs he could demonstrate were small petechial haemorrhages on the lining of the lungs, which occur when death is sudden. Apart from mild inflammation of the throat and upper respiratory tract, he could find no reason for her death. In particular I remember him saying there were no signs of disease in the lungs. In the circumstances, he recommended that specimens from various organs should be sent for further forensic examination, in case she had been poisoned. I heard no more, but a month later I rang the coroner's officer to ask if there was any further information as to the cause of death. I was informed that nothing amiss had been found to suggest poisoning, but on pushing my request for an actual cause of death, he said, "Oh, didn't you know. It was due to broncho-pneumonia." I found this surprising and disturbing. Having found nothing abnormal in the lungs, how could she have died of broncho-pneumonia, a disease usually associated with old people and having the nickname "old man's friend"? My faith in the post mortem room as the final arbiter in medical puzzles suffered a severe blow on discovering that it was no better than the rest of us when rationalising a cause of death, when in truth, none has been found.

And now two examples of "misses"; one rather tragic and the other highly amusing. In my early days in practice I had a patient, a young man who was a medical student at the same College from where I had qualified. I was happy to let him shadow me in surgery on occasions in order to give him added experience in his chosen profession. Years passed and he qualified and later entered into private practice with a number of theatrical types among his patients. One day he rang and asked a favour of me: he was expecting to see a Hollywood film star who was due to visit England over the following few days. Unfortunately he would be away, and would I see her in his absence. If I agreed, he would make all the necessary arrangements, and let me know when and where I could see her. I was happy to oblige (another example of receiving the gift of a patient being famous producing feelings of gratification). Two days later he rang with the devastating news that our patient had been involved in a car accident in the USA and had been killed. The news was later ratified in all the papers, as she really was very famous and is still remembered as second in the glamour stakes only to Marilyn Monroe.

The second case happened after I had been a partner in the practice for about a year and a local GP had died unexpectedly. He had, unfortunately, a very disturbed personality and although only in his fifties, was addicted to both alcohol and drugs, as a result of which his practice had been reduced to less than a thousand patients, who had remained remarkably loyal to him. As my own practice at the time was still quite small, I applied to take over the vacancy left by his death, and was successful. He practiced from a surgery just too far away to expect his patients to travel to my surgery, so I attended his surgery twice a day, to look after them. It was not a very busy practice and I always took a book with me to read during the quieter moments. I was reading the latest bestseller, when an elderly, smartly dressed man with a thick German accent entered and asked if I was the Dr Carne who had taken over the surgery. On answering in the affirmative, his next request rather flawed me. He asked if he could join my list of patients, and when I asked if there was any special reason he replied, "Yes, I have done a thorough research on you, and have discovered that you only just failed to get into Harley Street." I did not think it worthwhile to disabuse him of how the system works, and as I was building up my practice, I accepted that he probably meant it as a compliment, and after that we got on very well together.

To return to the theme of "myths". It was during the time I was closely associated with Michael Balint that I became aware of the "myth of the more powerful doctor". This myth is shared by both patients and doctors: we both believe that if we, personally, do not know the solution to a problem (or in medical terms, the diagnosis and/or treatment of a particular illness), some more powerful being "out there" will be able to provide it. This helps to understand why some patients make constant, but perhaps not unreasonable, demands to seek a second (or third or fourth) opinion, the request usually accompanied by the desire to see the "top man in the field". (The mind boggles at the thought of seeing a "top bottom man", and I was amused when on an official visit to the opening of a new Health Centre, I was introduced to the "head chiropodist"). From the doctor's point of view, it is difficult not to fall into the trap of believing there really is someone who will solve the puzzle that has alluded every medical person seen to date. If not controlled, this leads to condemning the patient to a permanent round of referrals and investigations, with consequential fixation on the unexplained "illness": it can be argued that sometimes this is more dangerous than missing the diagnosis. One of the arts in practising medicine is to know when to stop. Perhaps it is also part of good writing to know when to stop, so I will conclude this chapter now, unless there is a more powerful writer out there who knows better!

CHAPTER VIII

From Prime to
Paracme – Passing Thoughts

I recently came across the word paracme. It is new to me, and probably to most people as it is not to be found in the dictionaries one usually has in the home, but it is in the *Complete Oxford Dictionary* (20 volumes thick) and perhaps of even greater authenticity, it can also be found in the book of "Official Scrabble Words". As the latter has no definitions, one needs to go to the Oxford Dictionary to find that it is defined as "the point reached at which one has passed one's prime". The trouble with this description of "that time of life . . ." is that it implies there is an end point; like the leaves of autumn, it can only happen once before they irretrievably fall to make way for a new birth. "Paracme" lasts for the rest of one's life, and long may it last!

All this, of course, begs the question "what is one's prime?" Professionally a doctor's prime, at least in the eyes of his patients, lasts for that very restricted time between "being too young and inexperienced" and "being too old and past it". My guess is that for most of us that is about the age of mid-thirties to mid-fifties, or if you have had a little luck, kept to a good diet and foresworn tobacco and alcohol, the early sixties. In this chapter I propose to relate some of the thoughts, teaching points and conclusions I reached before my paracme.

Breast - v - Bottle. During the time I was in practice, debate raged between the relative benefits of breast-feeding as opposed to bottle-feeding of infants. The merits of one against the other changed from time to time rather like the pendulum of a clock swings from side to side. I have always felt that neither one nor the other has sufficient benefit to outweigh the true wishes of the mother. Pushing for one against the other ignores the fact that women differ in their basic instinctual need and desire. What might be very fulfilling to one mother may be an unwarranted intrusion and onerous task for another. I have often been consulted by a mother whose attempt to meet the wishes of what she has been told is "best for her baby" has been thwarted by her own dislike of the process, or perhaps her failure to achieve success. The frequent consequence of this conflict is unconscious hostility to the baby associated with feelings of guilt, and a resentful, miserable, and very often hungry, baby. I coined the phrase: "a baby prefers a warm, loving bottle to a cold, rigid breast". This may not be popular in the present climate of favouring the breast, often expressed with missionary zeal, but I stand by my view. I accept that when all things are equal, there are advantages in breast-feeding, but the world is peopled by too many happy bottle-fed individuals (myself included) to discount the method entirely.

Disorganised to Organised Illness. I have written elsewhere of the influence Michael Balint had on the way I practised medicine: the next contribution also owes much to what he taught me. A patient presents to the doctor with a set of complaints, known as symptoms. The general practitioner, being the doctor of first contact, is presented with this package, rather like a box of Lego bricks. They have no definite pattern, but at the same time have the potential to be sorted into wondrous objects, if put together properly (but equally the potential for a ghastly mess if not). He called this "the disorganised illness that the patient brings to the doctor". He also likened it to a gift from the patient to the doctor. The doctor accepts the gift, but recognises that he has to make some sort of order out of the chaotic structure presented. In other words, the Lego bricks have been given as a loose mass of bricks and the doctor has been asked to make a structured model from them. At this stage it is important to remember that there is more than one structure that can be built from the bricks supplied. The doctor then takes on the responsibility of putting the bricks together in some kind of pattern and when he (the doctor) is satisfied, hands the package back to the patient. But it is no longer the disparate "disorganised" illness that he has been gifted, but a tight package, neatly tied with ribbon and given a tight knot, that can only be dismantled with great difficulty, or sometimes not at all. Balint called this "organised illness". The patient accepts the package, at which point it becomes his property: anyone who tries to take it away does so at his or her peril. Being their property, the patient puts his copyright on it, and now for example, describes the package or disease he has been given as "my arthritis", or "my migraine". The problem is that the diagnosis made may not be correct or may be capable of more than one interpretation. There may be a choice of therapies, but the patient is intent on keeping their property intact.

Let me give an example: a patient (X) has a headache and consults a doctor. Doctor A diagnoses "migraine": Dr B diagnoses "tension headache": Dr C diagnoses "? brain tumour". Depending on which doctor the patient has consulted they now own either migraine, tension headache or a possible brain tumour. If they then consult another doctor who makes a diagnosis different from the one that has been given, it is not uncommon for the doctor in this situation to find himself facing great difficulty if he tries to alter therapy or diagnosis (unless, of course, he is a "more powerful doctor" that has been recommended by friends or been found on the internet!)

Alcohol and the Individual. A quickie on alcohol intake. I do not intend to go into the pros and cons of drinking or its benefits and its dangers. Just a "thought for today" (or any other day): if you feel you need a drink, it is definitely the time not to have one.

Dependence and Independence. When discussing the relationship between doctor and patient, the importance of considering "dependence" and "independence" cannot be rated too highly. Much is written and read about "doctor knows best" and paternalism of doctors (a bad thing) and patient choice and independence (a good thing). These views should not be allowed to go unchallenged. The ideas were probably born while the originator was fit and well and sound in mind and body. It fails to take into account how one might feel if unfortunately finding oneself in a threatening situation. The often-repeated plea to be allowed to die in dignity is laudable, but how can we be sure it is also the view of someone who has reached the stage where this is not possible? Faced with a situation that is inevitable, it is quite possible that one's aspirations and hopes alter.

I do not pretend to know the answer to this conundrum, but I do have a theory about dependence and independence. Most of us prefer to be independent and make our own decisions, and although we often seek advice, the final decision and responsibility remains our own. However, when we are ill most of us happily accept dependence on another, whether that role falls to a health professional, family member or friend. The degree of dependence will in turn depend on the severity of the situation and our own personality. Dependence on the doctor is acceptable and can even be therapeutic, but on regaining one's health, return to independence is equally important. There is a danger in allowing the dependence to last too long, and a point is reached at which the good doctor has to give up the control he has on his patient, and encourage the return to independence. Sometimes, the gratification felt by the doctor from having the patient need him leads to his failure to recognise this fact, and too often one sees the deleterious effects of an overlong or continuing dependence on the doctor. Let me give an example. Observation of a young child playing in the park confirms that the mother, reluctantly, has recognised the child's wish for independence, and allowed him to run around unattended. Almost inevitably, the child falls over and although not badly hurt is likely to stay down on the ground, look round at its mother and if she is not paying attention, start to cry to draw her notice to his plight of being hurt and requiring attention. In other words, independence is forgotten and dependence is the order of the day. Mother, recognising the crisis runs to pick up and comfort the child, who once reassured that there is no serious hurt, wants to return to running around and playing. The wise mother allows this to happen, but it is not unusual that mother, in her desire to insure that her infant is not hurt any further, wants him to stay by her side. In these circumstances it is not surprising that a feud develops between parent and child, which usually the child wins, but not without a great deal of negative feelings between the two. My theory is that an ill patient is like the child: while ill they want "mummy doctor" (is maternalism as pejorative as paternalism?) but once better, a healthy patient wants "mummy doctor" to retreat into the background. Sometimes, dependency provides gratification to the patient, who then needs encouragement to return to independence and good emotional as well as physical health. The art of good medical practice is in recognising when this point is reached. Too soon (as so often happens nowadays with early discharge from hospital) and the patient regresses; too late and a kick-start may be required, the doctor having to weather the anger this may initiate.

The Patient Who Makes The Doctor Angry. It will probably be denied by some doctors that they are ever angry, but those with personal insight may find these thoughts of interest. As long ago as 1976 (37 years at the time of writing and it seems like the week before last!) I wrote an article for *Mims* magazine under this title as part of their "Behaviour in General Practice" series. I described the feeling as being like a battlefield, with the doctor and patient being the warring factions. I have recently re-read the article and in spite of passing time making some of my conclusions no longer topical, I think some are worth repeating.

I likened the anger that might threaten a consultation with various wars in history, depending on the degree of anger involved. The most damaging I likened to World War I. It described those doctors who appear to be at permanent war with their patients, or patients with their doctors. Included in the war was "the system as a whole", but in particular the NHS, neither of which could do anything right. As with other world wars, only total surrender can end the fight, something that neither the doctor nor patient can contemplate. The likely outcome is for the doctor to be killed in action (resigns from the profession) or deserts to other pastures where he hopes the grass will be greener (goes abroad).

Also included were lesser degrees of warfare including "the fifth column" or the enemy within. This described the fight between hospital consultants and GPs: perhaps less present today than in the past, but still smouldering in some areas. Some of the anger, it must be said, has shifted towards the politicians who nowadays feel they are the Messiahs of the service and are the only ones who know what is needed, and "you'd better do as we say".

Next was the war that nobody wins. At the time I called this the Vietnam War, but today it would be the Afghan situation. This refers to the patient who can never be satisfied and his expectations never met. Instead of re-examining the options offered by the patient, or the patient accepting limitations to the magic that the profession can supply, both continue to be dissatisfied with each other, as a result of which little is ever achieved.

"The Pyrrhic victory" is when either patient or doctor (or both) firmly believe they are the victors and their views have been accepted by the opposite party, though in fact, they are so firmly entrenched in their ideas that neither has really given in and the unproductive situation deteriorates even further.

Revolution describes the patient who finds it impossible to accept the rules and conventions of the consultation. If the doctor runs an appointment system (the idea was quite new in 1976), they always want to be seen at their own convenience: if certificates can only be issued under specific circumstances, they will want one anyway. The apotheosis of the medical revolutionary is the patient who insists on a home visit out of hours, especially at night, for trivial medical reasons. The Balint research group who produced the book *Night Calls* tried to research the reason why such calls were made, by agreeing to sit down and have a "long consultation" with the patient when called out at night. They hoped to come to an understanding of the underlying agenda. They had to give up the project, because they realised that in many cases they were much too angry to carry out the research.

The Cod War described the situation with Iceland at the time when we were very angry with each other over fishing rights in the Atlantic and North Sea, but liked each other too much to let it disturb our relationship outside of the specific issue of fishing. The scenario of an underlying, smouldering anger, which both parties have learned to accept, is perhaps more common in the doctor/patient relationship than is usually recognised. Relationships appear cordial, but mistrust remains.

Finally, I described a war that was just avoided, namely the situation at Munich in 1938. Neville Chamberlain announced "peace in our time" on his return from meeting Hitler. It only lasted a year before the true war exploded: in the surgery one sometimes wishes the peace could be maintained for as long as a year! One patient I remember, who fitted into this category, came in one morning and her opening remark was, "Let me look at your face". When I asked why (as she knew I would) she replied, "So that I can see how far I can go before you get angry with me." Another lady, with whom I was plagued over a period of at least 30 years, managed to make me angry on every occasion she consulted. On one occasion I failed to control my anger any longer and asked her why she continued to consult me when nothing I did was of any use to her. Her astonishing reply, stated coolly and politely, was, "But doctor, I always feel so much better when I leave you." My realisation that my function was to act as her punch bag did help me to cope with the situation with greater equanimity.

Patients, Doctors and Lawyers. Since retiring in 1998, my wife and I have become cruise enthusiasts. We like the smaller ships, carrying no more than 400 passengers, but they must be large enough for the comforts we have become used to in life. "Silversea" cruise ships fulfil all these functions admirably, and the passengers we meet on board have for the most part been most interesting as well as multicultural. On one cruise to China and Japan we spent a fair time with a delightful group from many different countries. On one occasion we found ourselves dining at the same table with passengers from five different points in the globe, namely Britain, Canada, USA, Mexico and Australia.

On another of our cruising holidays, we stopped over in Iceland and while there we joined about thirty fellow passengers, nearly all American, on a coach trip to see some of the country, including the hot springs and geysers, which are a feature of Iceland. On the way back to the ship, our driver dutifully stopped at a red traffic signal but the driver of a following large lorry, with hoisting equipment and concrete loaded on the back, did not think it was necessary. Consequently he smashed into the back of our coach, which fortunately was made of sturdy material. Although the back of the coach was flattened, the large, heavy vehicle did not actually enter the cabin of our bus. However, as anyone who has had a similar experience will know, it made a noise as if the whole bus had exploded under the impact. I felt that as a doctor I had a duty to do something, or at least check that no human damage had occurred. In addition my wife was jabbing me in the ribs saying urgently, "Do something" (as doctors' wives are prone to do). I spoke up: "I'm a doctor, is anyone hurt?" Not a word in response and I sat back reassured. Almost immediately, an American voice was heard: "I'm a solicitor, anything I can do?" Twenty voices spoke as one: "I think I've suffered a whiplash injury!"

CHAPTER IX

You've Got To 'Ave Art

When my wife and I first met, I was still at school and she had just started working as a secretary. Money was tight, but one day while wandering through the arcade at Swiss Cottage station (the arcade no longer exists though the station remains) we noticed a small shop, really a kiosk, selling what was advertised as antiques but was more realistically bric-a-brac. In the window was a small oil painting of the portrait of a young girl, in the style and dress of the period of Joshua Reynolds. She had a winsome expression, with an enigmatic smile that reminded us of her more famous sister, Mona Lisa. We fell instantly in love with her and after much bargaining and careful saving of money, we managed to purchase her for all of £6. We had no home of our own in which to hang her and for the next eight years she remained packed carefully in a suitcase. She now has pride of place in our dining room, and constantly reminds us of our first foray into the buying of antiques, and bric-a-brac, and (no doubt) some bric-a-brac disguised as antiques.

Although we knew in our hearts and minds that she was not likely to be a lost masterpiece, we did harbour some hopes that she might be. (Don't we all?) In 1959 we came across an article that explained how lost masterpieces could be reclaimed by having a free authentication by an expert at The National Gallery. We began to wonder whether she might, after all, be at least a minor masterpiece. If so, how would we spend the fortune that her sale would bring? The notion that we were already being disloyal to our beloved one only just managed to cross our mind before it was instantly banished. (If you are a regular lottery ticket buyer you will recognise the feeling of the euphoria every Tuesday and

Friday . . . before the reality of the actual draw on Wednesdays and Saturdays.) We made a joint decision to take her along for the authentication, our sense of greed overcoming any feelings of guilt. What we had not reckoned for was the fact that we were not the only ones who had read the article. Nor were we alone in believing that we were sitting on a hidden fortune.

We packed our little girl in newspaper and carried her in a carrier bag. This was a security measure to protect her anonymity on the Tube. On arrival at The National Gallery we were only marginally put off by the large queue of fellow authenticees, all carrying carrier bags containing newspaper- or brown paper-wrapped paintings of varying sizes. Great care was taken by everyone not to let anyone else see their valuable possession, although the occasional glance into their own carrier bag could be observed.

On arrival at the Gallery we were directed to a waiting room. This was an annexe to one of the larger galleries, and some paintings had been left hanging on the walls, just to remind us of what a real masterpiece should look like. Chairs had been placed round the walls, and it resembled a doctor's waiting room; the only difference being that the inhabitants' facial expressions were full of hope and expectation rather than the more usual look of anxiety. No one spoke to anyone else, and the air was filled with sepulchral silence. The only change of expression came when someone took yet another surreptitious peep into their bag, while everyone else watched with an air of contempt.

There were about thirty people in front of us (and very soon as many behind us too) but we were called in for our examination within about 45 minutes. A quick mental estimation meant that, unless there were several authenticators, which seemed unlikely, little more than a minute was being assigned to each valuation; perhaps equivalent to the inadequate five minutes per patient that was the average time then for a GP consultation. The sight of the authenticator, a short, insignificant-looking gentleman in corduroy trousers and sandals, did not assuage my fears. I had expected that someone at least equal to an auctioneer at either Sotheby's or Christies would be needed for such an important task, but he looked rather like the man that had sold us the picture. Had we come, heaven forbid, to a mere general practitioner, not a specialist?

As we entered, our expert had just completed his task of deflating another hopeful client, who in turn was shamefacedly repacking his treasured painting in its brown paper cover. He indicated to us to place our little girl on the table in the centre of the room (or was it an examination couch?). I could sense from his expression as he approached that he had already dismissed our offering as being commonplace, but was kind enough to say that she was "very sweet" and possibly a portion from a larger painting. There was no indication as to who might have painted her, but he was certain it was by an unknown. He gave us no time for questions but called for the next client and we were left to pack up and go. The similarity in my mind between the circumstances in which we found ourselves, and a visit to the doctor, brought forth an anguished plea of "Can't we have a second opinion?" But he was gone and we were left to return home with our painting. Many years have passed since then, and we still love her; indeed, have grown even closer to her. And who knows? Perhaps he was wrong . . .

In the early 60s, Pearl and I were on holiday in Sussex and while there we were browsing through an antiquarian bookshop. We noticed hanging on a wall situated at the side of a dark, rather rickety staircase, a small painting of Venice. It had probably hung there, unrecognised, for many years. It was nicely framed with a brass plaque stating it was by Francesco Guardi, one of the two famous Venetian artist brothers. They lived at about the time of Canaletto and apparently the numerous small souvenirs they painted were sold to visitors to Venice in much the same way that postcards are sold today. On questioning its provenance we were informed by the owner of the shop that it had previously belonged to John Christie, the owner of Glyndebourne near Lewes, where operas have been performed in the magnificent gardens every year since the 1930s. It was priced at a ridiculously low figure by today's standards – £75 – but a sum that was not quite so low then. It was certainly a lot more than we could afford to pay. But it was lovely, and with the added allure of its possible investment value, we took a deep (deep) breath and bought it.

Once more, discretion failed to be the better part of valour, and curiosity made us want to research whether we had acquired a valuable asset, or merely a copied foundling. Accordingly we rang one of the famous auction houses who advised us to bring it along for an assessment. First signs were very encouraging: it looked as if it could be genuine and the provenance was good. They said they would like to research it further and asked us to leave the painting with them. It actually took three months before they would commit themselves to a definite opinion. To our great disappointment they concluded that it was unlikely to have been painted by the great man himself, but, they assured us, it was "a very nice painting". For the money we had paid, this wasn't enough; I wrote to the gentleman from whom we had purchased it, and told him that the auctioneers had come down against it being a genuine Guardi. "In the circumstances," I informed him, in a rather high-minded manner, "you may like to buy it back from me at the price I had paid." Maybe his immediate response, agreeing with my offer, should have alerted me that he had other ideas about its authenticity, but I only felt relief that I had saved £75. Looking back on it now, we regret not keeping it. It looked lovely on the wall, and had become a major talking point among our artistically minded friends. Whether genuine or not, the price we paid would seem very cheap now.

Discerning readers will have recognised that our taste in art is traditional. We have collected some Victorian watercolours over the years, and I really do not understand or enjoy so-called modern art (with some minor exceptions). In 2008 we were in Venice at the time of the Biennale and took the opportunity to visit it. We spent an interesting and instructive morning browsing the various pavilions, some of which were very much better than others. One pavilion in particular stands out in my mind. It was very modern and imposing, the theme being glass and mirrors. One exhibit was a small room made of glass walls and windows. One window was composed of two large panes of glass, an upper and a lower frame. The upper frame had a spider-like crack in the glass running right across it, and this was mirrored on the bottom pane, producing an artistic pattern. I had the temerity to ask the person in charge whether this pattern of cracked glass was an artistic statement or an accidental breakage. He was honest enough to tell me that the upper frame had been dropped and cracked during installation so the designer had carefully reproduced the pattern on the lower frame: most people, he told me, complimented the designer on his artistic genius.

*

"Caveat emptor" (buyer beware) is a well known legal warning. Sometimes one has to remember that "seller beware" can be equally important.

If you lived during the winter of 1974 you will remember it as "the winter of discontent". Power cuts were not uncommon and I was attending a Balint research group, which at that time was held at University College Hospital in Gower Street, and was later to produce the book *Six Minutes for the Patient*. In walking from Warren Street station to the hospital I took a short cut through Maples. This was a large traditional departmental store, but like so many others was in the throes of shutting down to make room for a more commercial property. A power cut was on and the only lighting in the store came from a few very dim emergency lamps, supplemented in some departments by candlelight. As I was early for my meeting I wandered up to the fourth floor, where the antique department was situated. I was surprised to find they were holding a huge closing-down sale, but unfortunately the only items in which I was interested were out of my financial range. Lurking in a dark corner I saw a delightful oil painting on wood.

Even in the dim light, it looked superb, and I gleaned from the assistant, who had noticed my interest, that it had been brought up from their basement store room where it had languished for goodness knows how many years, in order to be sold off before the store shut for good. There had not been time to research the painting properly so it was being shown as "in the style of Van Goyen"; though they thought it possible it was actually painted by the artist himself. Jan Van Goyen was one of the old masters of the 17th century. His paintings in the 1970s fetched upwards of £30,000. Here, the price being asked was £800; above what we could afford, but very tempting. After much thought, I persuaded my wife that, as well as a lovely painting, it might also prove to be a great investment. The gamble of purchasing it overcame our natural prudence, so we took a deep breath and bought it, successfully negotiating a small discount on the asking price. The painting was a typical Dutch scene of wherries sailing into port, and we took great pride in hanging it on our wall at home.

At first we adhered to the advice given, when purchasing antiques, to buy only if you love something and not because you may have made an investment. After about a year, however, we succumbed to temptation and wanted to know if we had bought a bargain or just a lovely painting. We sought the advice of one of London's leading dealers, who specialised in Dutch art, and were very excited when he visited us, took the picture off the wall and after careful scrutiny announced that it had all the elements of being genuine; he would like to research it further. This involved us having to obtain a colour photograph done by a professional photographer, and sending the photo to a Dr Beck in Germany, who was the world's authority on Van Goyen. In the meantime he advised us to insure the painting in the sum of £1,500. About two months passed before we received any reply. In Dr Beck's opinion, the painting was not by Van Goyen himself, but was probably painted about a 100 years later from an original etching, which was now housed in the Musee des Beaux Arts in Brussels. This was a little disappointing, but we were happy that the painting had a good provenance. A year after this, we were actually in

Brussels and went to the museum in question to research the original, but were informed that a superficial search did not show that they housed an etching of that nature. If we wanted to research it further, the fee would be very high. We continued to enjoy the painting and basked in the envy of our friends, none of who could boast such a fine painting which, just might still be ascribed to a master.

A further year passed and we were in the fine art department of a London store when we got engaged in conversation with the gentleman in charge of the paintings and etchings on display. We told him of our experience and our mild disappointment, and he buoyed our spirits again by informing us that we had not yet heard the last word on the subject. He offered to send a friend of his who was an expert in paintings of the period, having worked for several years in the valuation department of one of the large auction houses, to give us his opinion as to origin and possible value. We accepted his invitation, and a very nice gentleman visited us, took the painting down from the wall, and after an examination lasting all of a minute, stated unequivocally: "This is rubbish. It was painted at most a hundred years ago. You'll be lucky to get £150 for it."

I am almost ashamed to say that our first reaction was to blame the picture for our disappointment: as if it, and not us, had been responsible for our rash purchase. On further reflection, we realised that we still liked the picture very much (note how it was devalued in our minds from previously having loved it to just liking it!) but ought to consider selling it and cutting our losses. As our original expert, the London art dealer, had valued it much higher, we turned to him for further advice; indeed, he had earlier told us that if we ever wanted to sell it, he would be happy to act as our agent for a fee of 10%. He took on the consignment – and at this stage we learned some of the tricks of the trade.

He said he would put it up for auction and try and get it catalogued as a "J. Van Goyen". He explained that in catalogues

"Jan Van Goyen" indicated that it was painted by the artist himself; "J. Van Goyen" indicated it was speculative but might be by the artist; "Van Goyen" meant in the school of the artist: finally "in the style of Van Goyen" meant just what it said. To our delight he managed to have it catalogued as "J Van Goyen", but told us that it might be a few months before it came up for auction. He kept possession of the painting, and assured us he would inform us when the auction was to take place so that we could be present and enjoy the excitement. He also advised us to put a reserve of £1,500 on it. That figure again!

After about four months, having heard nothing, I asked our dealer friend if he had any news as to when the auction would take place. He told me he still had no news. After this, I rang about every month only to be given the same information. After a further six months, I rang and on this occasion the message was different:. Hadn't I heard? The auction had taken place the previous week and the painting fetched £1,500. I was flabbergasted. Not only had we lost the opportunity to watch our beloved painting being sold, but the figure was exactly the same as he at first valued it, the same as he had advised us to insure it for and the same as the reserve price. Other than ringing the auction house and ascertaining that it had actually been submitted to them and been sold for the price we had been told, we could only accept the dealer's cheque for the amount obtained, less the 10% commission. We had, in fact, doubled the amount of money we had paid, so had no cause for grumbling, but to this day we still harbour a nasty doubt that something about the whole transaction was not quite right. Did the gentleman who discarded the painting as "rubbish, worth no more than £150" hope that we would sell it to him and then make the profit on it? Was our dealer part of some sort of ring, in which dealers were in collusion? If so, did our dealer feel he could re-sell it as a genuine Jan Van Goyen? Did it now reside in a stately home – even a museum? So many questions. The hurt lives on. Seller beware indeed!

CHAPTER X

Per Ardua Ad Astra (I)

During my student and early professional years, National Service was an established fact of life. Studying medicine provided deferment from call-up until after qualification as long as one had been accepted at medical school. For my final two years at school studying for what are now known as A-levels, and which gave exemption from having to do the first year of medical studies, I lived in the blissful situation of believing I had been accepted at the Middlesex Hospital and deferment would be automatic as long as I passed my exams. Unknown to me was the fact that they had ignored the injunction to accept only 10% of pupils from school, leaving spaces for returning servicemen from the war. The elation of receiving my successful results in August 1947 was soon shattered by a letter from Middlesex Hospital to tell me that because of this regulation, they could no longer offer the place they had promised. To add insult to injury, they only offered that they would "view sympathetically any application I might make after my time in the forces". No guarantee was promised, adding to my depression. With only two weeks to go before term was due to commence at university, I thought any chance I might have of getting into medical school elsewhere must be very slim indeed. My girlfriend was more optimistic and insisted I write to all the London medical colleges, asking if they still had any vacancies. Fortunately, and not for the first time in our life together (we have since been married for over 60 years), she was right. Although the replies I received were as expected – "Sorry, full" – the London Hospital said they had one remaining interview session left, and I was invited to attend. "When were you informed your promised place had been taken away?" I was asked at the interview. I said, "Last week", to which they replied: "Didn't give you much time, did they?" They were obviously sympathetic to my predicament and it transpired they had kept back two places for school entrants; I was offered one of them, the other, I later discovered, going to a candidate in the same position as myself. As it transpired, the forced change was fortuitous, since the teaching at the London Hospital at that time was superb.

Being a qualified doctor gave an added advantage on entering the forces. One had automatic officer status and rank with guaranteed promotion to the next rank after one year. The year I qualified, 1952, was the last in which one became fully registered without having to spend a year in a pre-registration hospital job, which meant that those graduating up to and including 1952 could enter the forces immediately after qualifying; by 1953, one had to spend at least a year in a hospital job prior to being called up. The consequence of this was that there was a large hiatus in those eligible to be called up in the year that I qualified, leading to a shortage of service medical officers. Although normally deferment was granted to those wishing to increase the time spent in hospital training this was not so in 1952 and 1953. In order to overcome the shortage of available doctors, regulations became very much more strict and unless you could find a suitable job immediately, you were called up. In my case, after a six months job at my alma mater, I applied for an anaesthetic post, a specialty I was interested in at the time, but as I was unsuccessful in obtaining the job, I was told I would be called up within the next three months.

It was late in 1952 at the time; I spent the intervening two months doing locum hospital work over the Christmas holidays, and a two weeks locum in general practice in Dover. This was really my first experience of general practice and there is no doubt I was pushed in at the deep end. I had no car – was not even capable of driving one – and travelled by train to Dover with a briefcase containing the only medical instruments I possessed, a stethoscope and a combined auriscope/ophthalmoscope. As long as any prospective patient had a condition of the lungs, ears, nose, throat or eyes, I was fully equipped to deal with them. For any other condition I would have to rely on taking a good history and carrying out a full examination. A very good training for the next 42 years spent in general practice!

In Dover I stayed in the house of the GP who was away, looked after by his housekeeper, who must have been the world's worst cook. I still remember with a sense of nausea the smell of slowly cooking lamb chops that took two hours on a very low light to become edible; even then they weren't. The practice was a dispensing one and I remember the GP's final words to me before he left. "You won't have any trouble with prescribing – there are three bottles of medicine in the surgery. The white mixture is for stomach disorders, the black for coughs, the red for anyone who needs a tonic. Oh, and if they complain that the pain is severe, try giving them the pink aspirin." The only problem I had was with one patient who had been given a tonic at another practice that had been green in colour. It took a good deal of persuasion to convince him that "red tonics were the stronger of the two". The cough medicine, particularly popular, was described by the patients as the "strong one with the paregoric in it."

I was surprised to find that many of the inhabitants of Dover seemed to have chronic ear infections and subsequent deafness; so much for sea air being good for the respiratory system. One patient of whom I still have vivid memories was the local fishmonger. His shop was some way from where I was staying and required the local bus services to get to his home, which was above the shop. The view overlooking the sea was delightful, but I realised as soon as I saw him for the first time that he was in the terminal phase of cancer (I think the primary was in the lung). Medically I could do very little but he required twice-weekly injections of neptal to keep down the fluid retention that was causing severe swelling of his legs. This was the standard therapy for oedema (oral diuretics only being developed about ten years later) necessitating twice-weekly visits to give deep intramuscular injections. While visiting I found myself spending some time just talking to him, in the process learning something about running a fish shop. I was pleasantly surprised when during the latter half of the second week a delivery boy appeared at the house with a present of a large fresh lobster from my new friend. This was my first experience of lobster, but unfortunately the housekeeper managed to ruin it in the cooking. It was also my first lesson in the therapeutic benefit of just being a good listener. (". . . and comfort always.")

In the last two weeks left before joining the RAF, I did an intensive course in learning to drive, and managed to pass the test after only two weeks tuition; I must admit it was easier then than it is now. As I was not in employment and therefore not earning any money, I saw no reason why I should pay whatever the amount was for National Insurance. The only way you could be exempt from paying was to sign up for unemployment benefit, or as it was known then, the dole. I attended the local centre and dutifully gave my name and other details to the rather lugubrious gentleman behind the glass barrier. Eventually he came to the question, "What's your usual job?" I replied, "I'm a doctor." He replied dubiously: "Oh yes, a docker," examining my rather frail figure. "No," I corrected him, "a doctor." At last the penny dropped. "We don't normally get the likes of you registering here. There are plenty of jobs available if you want to work." Eventually I explained my position and he became much more understanding. In an attempt to be helpful to "one of her Majesty's boys ready to fight for Queen and Country", added the advice: "You know, if you continue to pay for the stamp [the means by which one made the required contribution to welfare], when you retire you will have accrued a larger pension. And if you die, your widow will receive a larger pension." (I was 24 years old and had been married for only nine months!) Even this tempting offer did not deter me from believing that the £3 a week benefit – not forgetting the exemption from welfare contribution – was too attractive an offer in my impecunious state to turn down. It took me about 25 years to realise he was correct and the advice was good. Fortunately, during one of the numerous reforms to the running of the NHS – these reforms so beloved by successive governments, but ruinous, in my opinion, to the service as a whole – I could buy "back years" with an interest-free loan in order to bring my pension payment up to a maximum. I am now reaping the benefit of this generous offer.

In February 1953 I left my wife (then six months pregnant) to join the service I had chosen. I was strongly reminded of the First World War song sung in similar, but more deadly, circumstances. "We don't want to lose you but we think you ought to go." I promised my wife I would try to find accommodation for us as soon as possible – after I had completed the one-month of service training, and had my posting.

During this first month we were asked if we would like to extend our compulsory two years into three- or five-year 'short-term commissions'; even consider applying for a permanent commission. Having weighed up the financial advantages in taking a short-term commission, I said I would accept their offer, but was told it was not for me to accept, but to apply and they would then decide if I was suitable or not. At the interview for acceptance I was asked if I had considered a permanent commission. I made the mistake of giving an honest, but not very tactful, reply that I would not consider a career in which if I achieved the ultimate success, the highest rank as a medical officer that I could achieve was Air Marshall, whereas if I was in other branches, I could become an Air Chief Marshall or even Marshall of the Royal Air Force. In spite of their shocked looks, I was forgiven and accepted as a regular rather than a mere national serviceman.

One final action had to be taken before I was fully accepted. As a regular officer, I had to have a "number one", or full dress uniform, for such things as official occasions and mess nights. We were given £100 to kit ourselves out, a large sum of money then. (Normal uniform was supplied free of charge.) I had the bright idea of buying my uniform as cheaply as possible, and after research found the cheapest option was at the Edgware Road Misfits Shop. As its name implied, they specialised in selling cheap clothing, "seconds" or items that had been rejected by discontented customers. A galaxy of uniforms for all the services and in nearly all sizes could be purchased, and at a fraction of the true cost. I had mixed feelings when the first one I tried on fitted like a glove!

I was now all equipped and prepared to spend the following three years "per ardua-ing ad astra-ing" – *Per ardua ad astra* is the motto of the RAF – and serving my country as a loyal officer.

CHAPTER XI

Per Ardua Ad Astra (II)

Of the three services, army, navy and air force, the latter was the one that I was most keen to join. I had reached the giddy heights of corporal in the Air Training Corps (ATC) at school, and during the early years of the war, when I was between the ages of 12 and 14, I had looked with envy on the RAF pilots in training who strutted around in their uniforms distinguished by a white band across the front of their forage caps. I did not realise then the horrors from which I might have been saved by being too young to be one of them. I belong to what might selfishly be thought of as the 'lucky generation': we were too young to fight in world war two, but too old now to be involved in armed combat.

It therefore came as a disappointment when my call-up papers came, ordering me to report for the army. This was not why I had spent hours with the ATC and several weeks attending an RAF photoreconnaissance station and a naval air base in Somerset as part of our training. With the confidence (some would say cheek) of youth, I wrote to the Ministry of Defence informing them of my own wishes and, rather to my surprise, received a letter back stating that my request would be granted. I was to join the RAF. The appointed date was the 1 March 1953 and I joined several other young doctors to commence an interesting and fruitful three years of my life.

One of my companions was Paul Freeling, who I had last seen as a seven-year-old pupil at the primary school we both attended. Our paths were later to cross at Balint groups and then at the Royal College of General Practitioners (RCGP), where Paul became one of its more famous teachers and a great influence in the training of general practitioners. Sadly, he died while still in the prime of life, but his memory lives on through a prize in his name awarded each year by the College.

During our preliminary month of training we were asked to state our preference for which branch of the RAF we would like to serve. After some thought, I concluded that the best postings might be with Coastal Command, with the benefit of living by the sea appearing most attractive. I was not too surprised to learn that I had, in fact, been posted to Maintenance Unit Headquarters (HQ). Although probably the most mundane of all the branches, the upside was that headquarters were situated in a purpose built building with good living accommodation for a single person, and because many of the personnel were staff officers of high rank, a batman (a personal servant) was provided and the food was excellent. As I was relatively recently married and my wife was pregnant with our first child, these benefits were not entirely appreciated by me, but shortage of housing made trying to find living quarters where we could be together impossible. A further problem resulted from the hiatus in available medical officers to which I have referred in a previous chapter. The HQ had until very recently been medically looked after by a part-time general practitioner who practiced locally. The medical needs of the unit were minimal and this had proved to be entirely adequate. About two months before I arrived, an RAF medical officer had been slotted in there, presumably to act as a reserve of medical personnel as the total numbers decreased over the following year. I became 'slottee' number two; now two of us were doing the work previously carried out by a part-time local GP. To our surprise, one month after I arrived a third medical officer was posted to the unit while awaiting an onward posting. For young men used to the heavy workload of being junior house doctors, the lack of available work was relaxing but very frustrating. After a further two months, the third to arrive was given a posting to a maintenance unit in Shropshire. As a young unmarried man, being so far away from his friends in London was not attractive, and being aware of my desperation to find accommodation where I could be together with my wife, he informed me that he had heard that accommodation was absolutely no problem in Shropshire; if I would swap the posting with him, I would have the opportunity to be with my wife in no time at all. It was only after I arrived at the unit, which was situated in the heart of the country, that I discovered that accommodation was nearly as difficult as it had been at headquarters – but without the benefits of a batman, and excellent food.

Recognising I might have been duped added to my frustrations, but within a very few days the adjutant informed me that he had heard of a possible flat that might be of interest to me. I jumped at the chance, and on researching the accommodation I discovered that it had an interesting history. The flat was situated in the wing of a local stately home, which was owned by one of the most noted families in England. (The double-barreled name of the retired brigadier owner was a combination of two names historians would immediately recognise.) The main Hall, named after the village in which it was situated – or was the village named after the Hall? – had been used as an army hospital during the war and the Brigadier and his family had moved into the old servants' wing, adapted to his own high standards of living. His butler and housekeeper wife and their family occupied the lower floor of the wing. The Brigadier, by now divorced and alone, had moved back into the renovated Hall leaving his flat empty. He had offered this flat to the Air Force if anyone was interested in renting it; and I certainly was. To add to the benefit, by the time I became 25 (then only a few months away) I would be eligible for marriage and living accommodation allowance. The Hall, as it was called, was situated in a large ornamental garden with five lakes, which in turn was open to the public every Sunday in return for a fee. The flat itself was large, comfortable, and had beautiful views over the Shropshire countryside with Wales just visible on a clear day in the distance. The butler, who lived in the flat below, had a daughter of 12 who was an ideal baby sitter if we wanted to go out. The only downside was that there were 72 stone stairs up to the flat, which was rather a drag, especially in transporting our baby daughter and her pram.

The next few months were idyllic. Although the medical work I was doing was rather routine and sometimes boring, it was the first time in over a year of being married that we were together as a family. In addition the flat was large enough to invite members of our family to stay with us, and we very quickly became members of the village community. The local GP introduced us to point-to-point racing, and a family friend owned the large Granada cinema in nearby Shrewsbury. We were given season tickets to go whenever we wanted.

Everything has to end, and after nine months of enjoyable living (although by this time we had both recognised that country life was not really for us) I made the elementary mistake of inviting the senior regional medical officer (SMO), who was attending the station on a routine inspection, to stay with us. "We have plenty of room," I told him, "and the flat is delightful." He accepted our invitation to visit for dinner (but not to stay) and after one look at our living accommodation I could see the expression in his eyes. Quite clearly he was thinking: "This is not for a national serviceman." (After all, to the regular officers, a short-term commission had the same lowly status as a conscript.) As a result within a month I found myself being posted abroad. The SMO was suitably apologetic, but "as I would understand, the contingencies of the service took preference . . ." However, recognising as he did that we were being put out (and, I suspect, rather liking my wife, as did everyone who met her), he said he would see to it that I got a good posting abroad. He had a friend who was stationed at the Air Ministry in London and was responsible for overseas postings. This was slightly reassuring since nearly everyone at that time was being posted to the Canal Zone (Egypt, Jordan and the Suez Canal areas). These places were not only very hot, but also no family members were allowed to be there. I did not like the prospect of another long period away from my wife and daughter.

I think when he made the promise of a comfortable posting he had not reckoned on my perseverance. Taking him at his word

I rang not once but on several occasions, asking him if he had done anything about my posting. Fortune came to my rescue: I happened to phone him just when he was with his friend who wielded the power of posting, and after a mumbled conversation on the other end of the phone, he returned to me and asked, "Would Malta be OK?" Ogden Nash, the famous humorous poet, whose work I recommend to anyone who is not familiar with it, once defined the word instantaneous as the "the time taken between a traffic signal turning from red to green and the man in the car behind you hooting". I think at that time in my life the word could be more accurately described as the time taken between his question being asked and my resounding "Yes!" down the phone.

I was pleasantly surprised when, true to his word, my orders for Malta came through. This involved a week's course in tropical medicine, and I felt very guilty when I discovered that not only were we all married, but only myself and one other, who had been posted to the Far East – heaven knows what influence he must have had – had been given postings to places where our wives would be able to come too. All the others had been posted, as I had feared to be, to the Canal Zone.

My next task was to research Malta; also how to make life as comfortable as possible while I was there. First I discovered that if you could provide an address where you would be living while abroad, your family could travel out with you. I was tipped off that a hotel counted as a residence and through a local travel agent I discovered a reasonable hotel and made a booking. (At that time Malta was not the fashionable and popular tourist destination that it is today.) I also visited the Jewish Board of Deputies for any names that I could look up when I got there. The secretary bought down an old tome from its shelf, dusted it down, and on looking up Malta discovered that the total Jewish population could be counted on two hands. However, one name he gave me was that of the President of the Jewish Community in Malta; we worked out from his CV that he would have been

90 years old. Not too promising! When I later introduced myself to him I discovered that he was, in fact, the son of the man in the book; his father, who had the same name, had been dead for some years. He was a jovial character, only a few years older than we were, and he introduced us to the "best fish restaurant in Malta"; also to my first experience of Italian wines. The local Maltese wines, although cheap, were rather rough, though they have improved since then.

Before leaving England for Malta, I met someone who had also been stationed in Malta and he told me of a family whom he had met, and who had been both charming and hospitable to him and his wife while he had been there. It turned out that they owned fashion shops in Sliema and Valletta and consisted of three generations that had settled in Malta from Austria as refugees, arriving just prior to war being declared. Their story was interesting, but rather frightening: desperate to escape from the atrocious regime in Austria, the eldest son had come to plead with the authorities to allow them in to Malta. This was an unusual request for Malta, but because they owned a millinery factory in Austria, which had used outworkers from Malta, he managed to persuade the Maltese government to allow them to settle there. To my knowledge, they were the only Jewish refugees actually living in Malta. Their daughter, who was to become our special friend, married an Englishman, a Mancunian, who was stationed in Malta during the war and had, afterwards, married her and stayed in Malta. They had two sons, the younger of whom was the same age as our daughter, by this time just over a year old.

Lisl, as we knew her, showed us wonderful hospitality and became a true and great friend. Her energy was boundless, and she was in a large part instrumental in ensuring our two years spent in Malta were so rewarding. In addition, over the next 30 years she helped make our holidays that we spent there, whether with her and her family or in later years at a hotel, the most enjoyable we have experienced. Sadly she died some years ago; we miss her very much. We also became friendly with her brother's family, who later came to live in England and became firm friends. Both he and his wife have died, too, but their children and grandchildren have remained close to us. After they came to England I looked after many of their medical needs, and I helped in the delivery of their youngest child, who is now a Professor of Dentistry and our personal dentist. Their older son has now risen in the legal profession to being a High Court Judge.

I also helped deliver their daughter's children. I had promised to be present, if possible, at the birth of her second child, but she was under the direct care of a consultant obstetrician. She went into labour on a Saturday evening, at which time I was attending a formal black tie dinner arranged by the BMA. The obstetrician had spent the day gardening and had still not changed out of his gardening clothes. We arrived at the hospital at about the same time, me looking very formal in black tie, and he in tattered pullover and wellington boots. It was very difficult for him to persuade the hospital staff that he was the one in charge, and I was there only to assist.

Having succeeded in persuading the Air Ministry that we were a family with accommodation in Malta, my wife, baby daughter and I travelled in an RAF plane to our destination. In those days planes were all propeller driven and jet engines were still waiting to be commercialised. It took upwards of ten hours to travel from Northolt Airport in London to Luqa in Malta, stopping at Nice on the way. Joanna, or Jo, our daughter, must have sensed something as from the time we got out of the car at Northolt until we arrived at Luqa she did nothing but cry. We landed in the early hours of the morning. The skies were blue, the temperature comfortably warm, and on many of the walls of the houses, the vivid blue of bougainvillea was prominent. A new section of our life was about to begin, and we felt confident that all would be well.

CHAPTER XII

Per Ardua Ad Astra (III)

When we arrived in Malta in the early hours of 27 May 1954, the only fly in the ointment was the knowledge that, when my time in the RAF came to an end, I would have to decide on a final career move. Short-term contracts and salaried partnerships in general practice as alternatives to a lifelong, full time commitment to partnership were not an option at that time to anyone with an ounce of ambition. I knew only too well that jobs were going to be hard to come by but I was firmly convinced that general practice was the road on which I wished to travel. Unfortunately, the year in which I would be released from the RAF, 1956, was a difficult one in which to try and enter general practice. The NHS was born in 1948 and under the regulations, before doctors became eligible for full superannuation (pension) rights, they had to serve a minimum of ten years, which meant, in effect, that no one in their right mind (and of competent fitness) would consider retiring until 1958. To compound the difficulty there was no upper age limit for doctors in general practice to retire. Hence I faced two years of a completely full market, before a glut of vacancies occurred as a result of a mass exodus of the older doctors. My wife and I considered emigrating to Australia, and I even applied for a possible "view to partnership" in the depths of mining country in the Welsh valleys. Much to my relief I was not even short-listed. A post in west London was advertised and looked promising, but I was not accepted. Many years later I met the GP who had rejected me at a rather prestigious meeting: a very nice man who blushed with embarrassment when I reminded him of the fact. He quickly overcame his embarrassment by looking me straight in the eye and saying, "Oh yes, I remember you well. The trouble was that you were too good for the practice." (Nice one, Charlie!) On the other side of the coin, while searching for a position, I did a two-week locum at a large health centre in north London. The principal was a doctor of the old school, and a gentleman in every sense of the word. Although I only worked for him for two weeks, he remained interested in my career until his own retirement about twenty years later.

In 1954 Malta was still an active military base, housing personnel from all three services plus the local Maltese army. In addition the Australian Air Force (RAAF) had an airport and base on the island and the Fleet Air Arm also had a station there. Malta itself is only about nine miles by 14 miles, but in addition there were two sister islands, Gozo and Comino, the latter lying between the other two larger and inhabited islands. Gozo was greener than Malta, as a result of which one had to contend with even more flies than on the main island. Comino could boast a blue grotto within a sea that was the bluest I have ever seen anywhere in the world. For a very small fee, one could persuade a local fisherman to transport you across from the mainland, together with picnic baskets, and then spend the day enjoying the sun and sea on this beautiful island.

Sometimes I have to remind myself that Malta, after tourism, development, independence and finally entry into the European Union, has changed almost beyond recognition. After our Air Force days we returned many times on holiday, and have observed these changes with great interest.

Malta had a population of about 500,000 in 1954, of whom over 95% were Roman Catholic. Traditional Catholicism was the normal way of life. The Church, and their attendant Clergy, had a very powerful influence on the behaviour and way of living of the resident population. In spite of being fiercely independent (and the war record of the nation's bravery and resilience is almost beyond belief; Malta had been awarded the George Cross for bravery by a grateful Britain) the vast majority accepted without question the doctrines of their religion and the interpretations put on it by what might be considered a rigid and conservative priest-hood. The cinemas showed mainly American and British films, but not only were they heavily censored over and above any censorship already imposed by the home authorities, the posters advertising the films were further exposed to censorship. A famous musical film of the time starring the pin-up girl of the 1940s and 50s, Betty Grable, was called *Bathing Beauties* and the poster pictured her resplendent in a bathing costume. Local censorship decreed that her arms and legs had to be blacked out so as not to show any naked flesh. Two-piece bathing costumes were not allowed to be worn in public. Malta has hardly any beaches so in consequence part of its attraction is the colour of the Mediterranean Sea, unblemished by the greying effect of drifting sand. Most of the coastline is made up of rocks and swimming is directly off these rocks, which has the additional benefit of mak-ing diving and snorkelling exceptionally appealing. Surrounded as it is by the sea, water polo and scuba diving were two pastimes at which the Maltese excelled. The governor of the island, a very important individual, looked after the British interests. A previous governor had been Lord Mountbatten who had by then gone to put his gifts into the more serious pursuit of transferring indepen-dence to India. It was an item of headline news in the local papers for some days when the governor's daughter thought that she could flout the convention of the country by wearing a two-piece bathing costume while sunbathing. She was wrong. She was arrested and spent some hours in the local police station before she was released, suitably humbled.

Nuns and priests, dressed in their traditional garb, were a com-mon sight in the streets, and the priests often carried umbrellas. This was understandable in the winter, but in the summer it never rained. (From June until September it was common practice to actually remove windscreen wipers from cars as they were super-fluous.) A rumour spread among the non-Catholic community that the umbrellas had a very definite purpose. It was believed that if after a year of marriage, a couple had not had any children, the priest would visit the young wife to give her counselling and advice on what we would call the behaviour "of the birds and the bees". In these circumstances he would leave his umbrella on the doorstep as a message to any husband who might be returning home – to tell him not to enter the house until the priest had left. The word was that this educative process had a practical hands-on (and maybe other-parts-on) aspect, as well as a verbal one. Priest and bride would be better educated after the session, and the beginning of a future family would be assured. I am sure there is no truth in the rumour, but it was not uncommon to see umbrellas on the doorsteps of some houses, even on hot dry days!

Although a small island, Malta was made up of many different towns, each with their own character. Each had at least one church, usually of cathedral proportions, with rich and beautiful interiors. Another oddity, which to my knowledge still exists today, was that every church that had an outside clock also had a second structure, looking like a clock but never showing the correct time. I was told the reason for this was to thwart the devil, who would be confused by the two different times and not, therefore, be in a position to enter the church during a service as he could never be sure whether the locals were at prayer or not. On the ubiquitous and colourful fishing boats an eye would be painted on the prow, to thwart evil and ensure safe sailing.

An interesting consequence of the religious influence was that every Sunday in summer a different town would celebrate their Saint's day. This involved a form of carnival, known locally as a *festa*. Townsfolk would dress in their Sunday best, stalls would be installed rather like small fairgrounds familiar to this country, many selling highly coloured sweetmeats (and I do mean sweet!). All the church valuables would be paraded through the streets accompanied by a slightly out-of-tune brass band and statues of the Virgin Mary and Jesus on the cross. It really was most impressive, but the climax of the celebration came in the evening as dusk fell. Collections would have been taken all year from the local population, many of whom could ill afford the contribution, in order that hundreds of fireworks could be bought and set off as a final climax to the day. Each town would vie with their neighbours to have bigger and noisier displays, and because of the proximity of each town to its neighbour, the fireworks could be heard (and often seen) all over the island. A wonderful sight, but the noise every Sunday could rise to horrendous proportions depending on how close you were to the *festa* of the day.

In the Malta we experienced in 1954, air conditioning was a rarity, television non-existent and refrigerators owned only by those well off enough to afford them. As I had reached the magical age of 25, when living allowance became available, the rent we had to pay for the flat we found (with the help of our new-found friend Lisl, who seemed to know everyone that was anyone in Malta) was subsidised. Officially I was also entitled to the use of a refrigerator, but none were available during the first months we lived there. Instead we were supplied with an icebox, which is, in reality, exactly that. Every two days the iceman would deliver two large blocks of solid ice, which fitted into the lower part of the cabinet containing the food, thus keeping it cool enough to avoid it going off too quickly in the heat. Eventually the RAF supplies officer took pity on us and said he had found a proper refrigerator in the stores, and he would have it delivered to us. Electricity and gas were not abundant enough to power our new acquisition and it was powered by paraffin. It was with great relief and anticipation that we lit the wick under the fridge and waited for it to cool to a suitable temperature. Unfortunately, the creation of coolness is accompanied by a surrounding heat gain and to our horror, as the back of the fridge warmed up, about two hundred cockroaches that had been happily lodging there evacuated themselves into our kitchen. Safari-like, we hunted them and crunched them out of our lives; but this is not one of our happier memories of Malta.

Shortage of water, both for domestic and drinking purposes, was a further problem to contend with. In later years investment into desalination plants made a huge difference, but while we were there what little water there was that could be drunk tasted foul and even if boiled for the purpose of making tea it would impart its thick, unpleasant taste into the tea. Bottled water was an alternative, but fairly expensive; there was a thriving local business of delivering crates of fizzy drinks. Yet another environmental problem that flowed from this water shortage was the care with which one had to use water for domestic purposes. It was rationed to one rooftop tankful a day; a meter ensured you paid for what you used. It cost ninepence (four and a half pence in new currency) for every flush of the toilet. You became used to sharing "your" chainpull with other family members. Believe me, you soon found out who your best friends were!

Good times rather than bad are more easily remembered and it is the long, glorious, but enervating hot summers that I recall rather than the sometimes stormy winters. Working only half days for two thirds of the time (only when on call did I have to work past 1pm during the summer months) meant I had time to enjoy family life.

As an officer, I was automatically a member of the Marsa Club, which had a private lido in Sliema and an open-air colonial type club with a golf course. Because of the dry hot weather, the greens were more appropriately referred to as the browns. In the clubhouse, al fresco dining and nights spent dancing under the stars form some of our happiest memories. Music was still truly romantic then; dancing a pleasant way to be close to your partner, although the American jitterbugging craze was creeping its way across the Atlantic, as everything American eventually does, and was soon to give rise to the Parkinsonian jerking that is nowadays called dancing.

Malta, at that time, had a large British service presence. Warships could be seen in the natural harbour at Valletta, for which Malta was so famous and where now even larger cruise ships have replaced them. Other smaller warships were anchored in the coves situated along the coast between Valletta and Sliema, where we were living. Later the famous and huge aircraft carrier, the *Ark Royal*, spent some time berthed in the dock, and we were fortunate to have an invitation to a cocktail party given by its officers on board. Naval hospitality was on show that night and it did not let the senior service down.

The main functions of the Royal Air Force were looking after the military side of the airport at Luqa, caring for the personnel passing through under the air casualty evacuation scheme ("casevac", of which later) as well as the medical needs of the families of the serving forces. The army cared for the specialist medical and obstetric needs and the navy for the surgical needs, each having its own hospital. In addition the local Maltese medical services could be called upon if needed.

Malta had its own medical college and teaching hospital and the standards were high, but the rather decrepit state of the hospitals were roughly on a par with some of those that we are familiar with in our present day NHS. Having said this, I am reminded of one episode in which the possible consequences might have been of some significance. I was approached one day by one of the Maltese clerks employed by the Air Force to help run the administration of the unit, who asked me if I could recommend a good pathology textbook to him. I told him that as a student I had used "Dible and Davey", a standard textbook at the time. He was scornful of my suggestion. "I've read that," he said, "I mean a large textbook." This aroused my curiosity a notch higher, and I asked him why he wanted to know. His reply shook me. "I am doing a correspondence course in medicine in order to become a doctor, at the University of Syracuse in Sicily." Not believing this to be possible (the months and years I had spent attending out-patient clinics and hospital wards, not to mention the gallons of midnight oil consumed, to achieve my own ambition could not, surely, have been totally unnecessary). I asked him: "But where do you do your practical clinical training?" "Oh," he said, "each summer I spend three months as an assistant to Professor _____, who is world renowned." I had never heard of him. "What branch of surgery does he specialise in?" I enquired. "Sex change operations," was his reply. This was 1955! As if he had not already astonished me enough, he then added: "While I will be there in the summer, he is changing twin sisters into twin brothers!' Perhaps nowadays I would not have been so surprised, but I had worked out that if and when he qualified, it would be under the auspices of an Italian University, which at that time was one of the few countries that enjoyed reciprocity with the UK, and he would therefore be eligible for full registration to practice in the UK. There is an epilogue to this story: about fifteen years later we were in Malta on holiday, and I saw an item in the newspaper that the Archbishop of Malta (still a highly prestigious and influential figure) had been ill, and his medical attendant had issued a bulletin on his health. The medical attendant was the man to whom I have referred above, who was obviously having a very successful career as a doctor. I should add I did not see any subsequent bulletin that the Archbishop had become the Mother Superior . . .

*

For my first year in Malta, I was stationed at Luqa airport. It had the dual role of being both a civilian airport (although a very small and quiet one) and a military one, which added to the interest. It also housed a small hospital (or perhaps more accurately a large sick quarters) for sick and wounded service personnel from the Middle and Far East and Africa, to be accommodated during a break in their journey by air, the so-called casualty air evacuation service. This is still operative but the standards today are much more sophisticated. Two nursing sisters were mainly responsible for the running of the unit, and from time to time we would play host to visiting dignitaries. Once we were visited by Prince Phillip, on another occasion by Lady Mountbatten. Both were very charming. There were sadder encounters, too. A young serving officer passed through. He had been serving in the conflict in Kenya between the Mau Mau, who were seeking independence, and the British; and he had developed poliomyelitis while fighting in the jungle, which had left him paralysed from the neck down. As was customary at the time, he was encased in an iron lung as his only means of breathing. About 25 years later, while watching a TV programme, I recognised one of the participants as the same young officer, who was still requiring artificial means of respiration and remained paralysed. I have an immense admiration for the capacity of some human beings to cope with adversity, but I also feel a great sadness at the necessity with which some people are forced to experience it.

Being stationed in Malta gave me the opportunity to purchase the first new car I ever owned. Hire purchase terms were extremely advantageous, and for a deposit of only £30 I became the proud owner of a brand new Volkswagen Beetle. Everyone in the officers' mess was curious as to its performance as so much had been written about it in the newspapers. It was decided after a discussion over lunch one day that there was only one way to find out how good (fast, really) the car actually was. The senior air traffic controller stopped all flights, landings and take offs for a period of half an hour, and I was dispatched in my car to the beginning of the runway. I was told to reach the fastest speed I could. In case I was tempted to cheat or exaggerate, stopwatches were supplied to check the actual speed. I am horrified to think that such irresponsible behaviour was allowed in those days, but I am sure that Jeremy Clarkson would have been proud of me.

While I was at Luqa, there was a very nasty air disaster. A civilian plane with nearly 100 passengers crashed on the island killing all on board. I was not on duty on that particular day and so was not involved in the rescue and recovery attempts, but many years later I was consulted in my practice by a woman who it turned out was still grieving over her son who had been killed in that very same crash. I told her I had been in Malta in the RAF at the time of the crash, and felt it would be helpful to add that I knew for certain that everyone on board had been killed instantly; it had been obvious that nobody had suffered pain. She found this very comforting, as I am certain most of us would in similar tragic circumstances.

Another incident made me realise, perhaps for the first time, that what patients understand you to say is not necessarily the same as what you thought you had conveyed. Research into this aspect of consulting has certainly confirmed this to be a fact; I found out the hard way. I was having lunch in the mess at Luqa, and an officer who had only arrived in Malta the week before spoke to me about his wife who, before coming out with him, had "suffered a mild nervous breakdown" from which she had fully recovered. But, he added, the change in climate and absence from her family was causing her to become rather nervous again and she was sleeping very badly. Would I, he asked, pay her a visit at home to reassure her that everything was alright? That she would soon settle down? And give her something to help her sleep? I explained to him that the responsibility for families at home was that of the medical officer stationed in Valletta. He was obviously in some distress, and was very persuasive, so eventually I agreed to look in on his wife that afternoon. He promised to be there. On arrival I found a woman who was not only mildly distressed but in the throes of what was a severe mental breakdown. It turned out that the "mild nervous breakdown" she had previously suffered was a fully blown depression and why she was allowed to travel out to Malta I cannot say. To add to the problem, my experience and knowledge of psychiatry was insufficient to cope competently with the situation, but each time I suggested a specialist should be called in both husband and wife begged me to give her a tablet to calm her down. After a good night's sleep, they were certain, everything would be alright again. "After all," they reassured me, "it has always worked before." After two hours of being unable to leave her, or to persuade her to attend the hospital, I allowed myself to leave a sleeping pill and to promise I would return the next day. On leaving, the husband said he would come with me as far as the shops as they had no supplies for their supper and he would buy her a steak and give her a good meal. Malta is always depicted as a sunny warm place with little rain, but this was in February when it can be very stormy indeed. This was such a day, with thunder, lighting and high, heavy seas crashing on to the shore. If it had been a film, one would have guessed that tragedy was just around the corner: and sure enough it was. During the 30 minutes her husband was out, his wife ran out of the house to the sea nearby (it is always nearby in Malta) and threw herself into the raging ocean. Her body was not recovered until the next day. Obviously there had to be an inquest. No blame was attached to me after the full history came to light, but I cannot forget the statement made by her husband to the coroner at the inquest. "I left her," he said, "only for a short time because the doctor had said she must have meat for her supper." I do not know what I must have said for him to have such a strong belief, but I still wonder whether the tragedy might not have ended as it did, if he hadn't misunderstood me and had stayed with her.

After I had served a year in Malta, there was a reshuffle of the medical contingent on the island. The officer who had been stationed in Valletta looking after the families was promoted to squadron leader at Luqa and his post became vacant. Knowing that my future was likely to be in general practice, this was an opportunity too good to miss. Looking after families full time was the nearest thing to being a GP and the experience would prove very useful. I therefore volunteered to take over his job, and was accepted, and moved out of the comfortable and supportive airport posting at Luqa into the more isolated and fully responsible medical posting in town. The site was a well-equipped health clinic with a nursing sister to assist me. We were responsible not only for the RAF families, but also the families of the navy and army. We also took our turn on rota duty, to look after the local Maltese army families, who lived all over the island. I was on out-of-hours call one day in three, which was quite strenuous. I was allowed to use my own car for home visits, for which I was paid a mileage fee. Although a small island, it was possible to clock up 70 miles of travel on one duty day because it was not unusual to travel out to a visit, return home, and soon after have to travel to another village on the island's outskirts. Another problem was finding the correct address once one had negotiated the way to the actual village (signposts were almost non-existent); then, having arrived at the village or town, one had to locate the actual house. The street would be named but the houses were not numbered; locals relied on houses having names. Given the religious nature of the island, a common name for the house was Mary's House; there might be three or four Mary's Houses in one street. I got round the problem by making for the local police station and giving them the name of the family. The likelihood was that one of the officers on duty would be related to one of the family and between us we would work out the correct house.

I was also involved in what must be one of the shortest postings in RAF history. The senior medical officer for Malta held the rank of wing commander, and a new wing commander arrived in Malta one Wednesday and marked his new posting by becoming blind drunk. Maybe he had left behind a bad experience in England and was glad to be away from it. Whatever the circumstances, for a reason best known to himself, he decided to seek out the most senior officer on the island – an Air Vice Marshall – and to tell him where to get off in no uncertain terms. He was given the choice of being kicked out the service, or returning to the UK as being medically unfit for service in Malta. Not surprisingly he chose the latter, and I had the delicate job of declaring him unfit so he could be packed off the island discreetly. I never heard of him again, and his replacement was a rather dull man who I have no memories of at all.

Although not as drastically as the short-lived Wing Commander, I nearly blotted my own copybook when I had to examine a Group Captain for his annual pilot's certificate. He told me proudly that he had been to a doctor while on a recent visit to the UK, who had told him that he had the blood pressure of an 18 year old. Foolishly I retorted, "And would you have been as happy if he had said you had the brain of an 8 year old?" My big mouth! Although he was without a sense of humour, he was not vindictive, so I was spared more than a threat that "it will take you a long time to reach high rank". As, at the time, I only had another year to serve, this threat was unlikely to affect my long-term career.

There is no doubt that our two years in Malta were made much more pleasurable by the friendship we had established with the Eders and Bergers (about whom I have previously written). Jews were rare in Malta, but there was a synagogue and services of a sort were held on high holidays, at which we all managed to get together. Lisl and her husband Sidney were extremely hospitable and on regular occasions had evenings at their home at which other Jewish service people would be present. One such was a civil engineer, who was a civilian attached to the navy. He held the equivalent rank of Captain and had been in the service for about 20 years. Outside of our little enclave, he kept his religion a secret as he felt this gave him more security. Another engineer, with whom over the years he had become very friendly, but who he had not seen for some time, had paralleled his career. He was pleased to receive a phone call from his friend to say he was visiting Malta on his way to a posting further afield. Could they meet up together? He gave the day when he would be on the island, but this coincided with the most important Jewish festival of the year, Yom Kippur, the Day of Atonement. Our friend took a big breath and felt that the time for sharing his secret had come. Diffidently he explained that he would love to meet up, but the suggested day was the one day in the year that he felt he should go to synagogue. Imagine his surprise when his friend responded, "Oh, are you Jewish too? So am I. I always felt shy about telling you." Friends for so many years, and neither had the courage to tell the other their hidden secret.

In the 1950s and early 60s Malta had a very large British influence: the telephone boxes were the pillar-box red that we were familiar with at home; the police in winter wore similar uniforms to our British bobbies; and English was the second language (almost the first). This influence remained into the later 60s, but when we returned to the island one year on holiday we noticed a big difference: the influence was no longer British, but very noticeably Italian. The reason for this change soon became clear. Whereas previously during the long, hot summers, it was the custom for the locals to sit outside their house watching the world go by, someone had discovered that by putting an aerial on the roof, Italian television could be picked up. No longer did one see people sitting looking out of their homes; now the chairs had been turned round and everyone was looking into the house at the newly acquired television. Italian became almost a second language, and fashion and *la dolce vita* became a way of life. Together with their emerging independence, Malta was no longer recognisable as we had known it – as an England away from home.

*

There is a toast that originated in the war and was relayed to me, rather incongruously, by my mother. She told me she had heard it from an RAF officer. It goes:

> *May you live as long as you want to,*
> *May you want to as long as you live.*
> *Bees do it and die,*
> *Kings and queens do it and sigh,*
> *But I can't do it, and I'll tell you why,*
> *I have a wife, to whom I have promised to be true,*
> *But I'll tell you what I'll do,*
> *I'll lie still, and let you!*

To me it sums up the bravado of the time; and perhaps it is tinged with regret at being born a generation too early to enjoy the freedom of the permissive society of the 1960s.

Those of you reading this that can remember the old film travelogues will be reminded of them when I write: "And so, I must leave the sub-tropical island of Malta and return to our native country, England." Malta and service life had come to an end, and the reality of facing up to starting a career in England beckoned. I accepted the £600 I had become entitled to for signing up to serve an extra year, and together with my "Edgware Road Misfit" dress uniform, and with Pearl and Joanna (soon to be joined by Debbie), our new life began.

CHAPTER XIII

Tuberculosis

Reading a short story by Somerset Maugham set me thinking about how things were during the period I was studying medicine and during my early years in practice. Comparing then with now makes one realise what enormous strides we have made, not only in medicine but also in all walks of life – although not all the advances have been entirely advantageous. There is an old story told of Mrs. Blotstein, a large, peroxided, Gucci-dressed and bejewelled lady, sitting on a plane when the lady next to her admires the enormous 20-carat diamond ring on her finger. "Yes, it is wonderful, but the only drawback is that it comes with a curse on it," she sighs. "Oh, what's that?" her new friend asks, and she replies: "Mr. Blotstein!" So it is with advances in medicine: one always has to be aware of the Mr. Blotstein that comes with every wonder cure or advance.

Somerset Maugham qualified as a doctor at St Thomas' Hospital, but became better known, indeed renowned, as a writer. The story about which I am writing is part of a miscellany entitled *Sanatorium* and it tells of life for a group of patients living in a sanatorium while suffering from tuberculosis (or as we knew it when it was very much more common than it is now, consumption or TB). With a true storyteller's skill Maugham describes how their illness, though an experience shared by them all, acts as catalyst to the way they react to their situation. The time it describes is probably the late 1920s or early 1930s, but although such institutions are rare today, they were still in existence (just) when I qualified. Segregation, rest and fresh air were about all that could be offered to sufferers of pulmonary tuberculosis (the commonest form), and their period of incarceration was anything from several months to many years; in some cases, life. The writer describes how they live a lonely, but comfortable, life, relying on each other for stimulation. They soon become expert at recognising each other's prognosis through the subtle changes in their looks, skin changes and energy levels. Friendships are made but so are enemies, and animosities and jealousies combine with support and care in their everyday life. Maugham describes how the two longest established inmates (eighteen and seventeen years respectively) argue over the privilege of who inhabits the "best room in the sanatorium", and devise as many ways as possible to irritate each other. There is a dramatic moment in the story when the older inhabitant, Mr. McLeod, achieves his life-time ambition while playing bridge: he succeeds in making a grand slam which has been doubled and redoubled by his opponents, one of whom is the other senior inhabitant, Mr. Campbell. Expressing his joy at achieving this goal, he slumps across the table, has a massive haemoptysis (bleeding from the lungs) and dies. This episode has major consequences, which act as the climax to the story. Mr. Campbell can now move into McLeod's room, which he has so long coveted, but finds he hates it and attempts, unsuccessfully, to move back to his old room. He never plays his beloved violin again, the very same violin with which he had annoyed Mr. McLeod over the years by his continuous playing. He has learned that he had relied for his emotional needs upon his old enemy and the loss was at least as severe as that felt by a spouse when a beloved one dies. Another consequence is that Major Templeton, a war hero stricken down with the deadly disease, whose numerous affairs with women had always been of a flirtatious nature and who had never before considered a serious relationship, decides that his love for the youngest patient in the sanatorium, Ivy Bishop (a pretty young woman of 29 who had spent the last eight years in various sanatoria, and who had become isolated from her family and friends who had found the burden of keeping up an emotional relationship with her too hard to bear), was deeper than any he had previously experienced. Against the advice of the medical director of the sanatorium, Dr. Lennox, to whom all patients looked for advice on how they should live their lives (a far cry from today's belief in "patient's choice", and how we view the concept of "doctor's orders" or "doctor knows best"), decides to live a short but fulfilling life rather than a longer but frustrating one: he proposes marriage, which she accepts and the story ends with them travelling off to their short but hopefully happy life together.

Another character in the story shows remarkable insight into the emotions experienced by someone finding themselves laden with a serious illness. Chester, who is an accountant in his 30s, married with children and leading a full and healthy life, is suddenly taken ill. Diagnosed as having tuberculosis he ends up in the sanatorium, where he realises that hopes of a cure are slight, and he is likely to die quite soon from the disease. Apparently well adjusted to the situation and getting on well with the other patients, he is allowed a visit from his wife at the end of each month. For the whole time leading up to the visit he cannot stop himself from talking about his wife, how much he loves her and how he can hardly wait for the time he can spend with her. Later in the story, his wife reveals to Ashenden (a regular character in Maugham's novels and acting in this story as an observer) that she cannot bear to visit her husband because he is so jealous of her good health and her ability to live the same normal life that he had enjoyed before his illness. Because of this, he takes it out on her in a verbally cruel way as she is the only person in whom he can confide his fear of dying and the unfairness of fate having chosen him rather than her to be ill. I suspect that this must be the true feeling of many of us stricken down with sickness; something rarely written about. Presumably Maugham's experience as a doctor gave him the insight to recognise this facet of illness. Eventually, Chester forbids her to come to see him, which she sees as a rejection, but in fact is because he has come to realise the effect his jealousy and cruel behaviour is having on her. The love he observes between Templeton and Ivy helps him to see that true love is worth sacrificing one's own selfishness for the benefit of the one who is loved, and he eventually confesses his true feelings towards his wife and the story ends with him telling her: "I want you to live and be happy. I don't grudge you anything any more and I don't resent anything. I'm glad now it's me that must die and not you. I wish for you everything that's good in the world. I love you." I have described this story at length because I believe it illustrates how sick people lived and accepted their role when I first entered the profession as opposed to the rather more selfish view that is prevalent now.

While a youth and young man, I was aware of such institutions for tuberculous patients, but the picture in one's imagination had a definite romantic ring rather than the truth of what it must have really been like to be ill for years of your life. Presumably many of these sanatoria were privately paid for, and therefore had a hotel quality about them. With the advent of the NHS, economics had to come into the equation of patient care. With the very real advances in treatment of tuberculosis, it has become a relatively rare disease (until its resurgence in recent years). Expensive sanatoria became redundant and were largely replaced by spas and health clinics, which are in the main situated outside Britain.

Although immunisation with BCG had first been shown to be effective in protecting against the disease over 100 years ago, when first used at the turn of the 20th century a rogue batch had caused an outbreak of the disease in children immunised with it in a district in Germany. As a result many people doubted its safety and as with the MMR scandal its general use fell into disrepute; 40 or 50 years passed and many lives were lost, before its efficacy and safety was re-established and the full benefits could be achieved. As a medical student one was exposed to the disease in hospital and it was therefore obligatory to be tested for immunity to the disease. At that time about 85% proved to be positive (protected against the disease and therefore not needing BCG) and only 15% unprotected. Of these 15% at least two in my year developed the disease and although by then treatment was more successful and they survived in good health, their education was delayed by at least a year. Now the proportion is reversed with around 85% at risk.

The pulmonary (lung) form of TB was the commonest manifestation, but it could affect most other organs of the body. Particularly vicious was TB meningitis, in which the bacillus attacked the lining of the brain and spinal cord leading to paralysis and brain damage. TB enteritis attacked the gut, usually from drinking unpasteurised milk from an infected animal (cattle had to be accredited as being disease free, but much milk that was drunk came from unaccredited farms). Another nasty form of the disease was when it attacked bones and joints leading to severe crippling. We rarely see these manifestations now except in third world countries, but I lived in the period where we still had to look after the remnants of the disease in patients who had been afflicted before prevention had become stabilised.

On a personal note, I had a cousin who was the only girl of seven siblings, and who developed tuberculosis as a young woman. It was at the time while I was a medical student, and when she became seriously ill with the disease a special consignment of streptomycin, a newly developed antibiotic and the first to be effective against the bacillus, was brought over from America. Unfortunately, used on its own, its efficiency is not that high, and it proved to be too little, too late. She died while still in her early thirties.

*

There have been many significant advances in medical diagnosis and treatment since my early days as a student and recently qualified doctor. I remember discussing at a cocktail party, with a professor of immunology, press reports that heart transplants "were on the horizon". He was insistent that it was not even a possibility, and went into a detailed scientific explanation of why this was so. Within five years the first successful human heart transplant had been performed. Now, although fortunately not common, it has become an everyday procedure. The problem has shifted from not being possible, to not having enough donated hearts to meet demand. Other major changes come to mind. Several diseases, considered to be death sentences in the 1950s, are now treated successfully or at least life has been significantly prolonged. Hodgkin's disease and certain types of leukaemia are examples. Although still posing a significant threat, treatment of many cancers has been greatly improved, although the argument remains as to whether screening of apparently healthy individuals is as useful as is made out by some authorities. Antibiotics have had an enormous influence in therapy but are in danger of being overused to the extent that their beneficial use is lost through the development of resistance. In more recent years the emphasis from too many antibiotics has perhaps been in danger of changing to too few. A potent argument has been put forward to avoid antibiotics in so-called "simple infections". Overall this is probably correct, but we must not, in my opinion, lose sight of the fact that having a low threshold for prescribing antibiotics in childhood infections may have been instrumental in the reduction of secondary complications. For example, we hardly ever now see diseases such as mastoiditis, chronic ear disease with deafness, bacterial endocarditis and nephritis, all of which led to severe consequences for the sufferer. From being untreatable, hypertension can mostly be controlled; ischaemic heart disease has been reduced in incidence, although not so far eliminated. Polypharmacy is now the pattern of therapy to the extent that side effects sometimes outweigh the advantages of treatment. The only problem with all these advances is that the NHS can no longer afford to look after the increasing and ageing population that results from it.

Finally, two epigrams come to mind, observance of which might benefit us all. The first is attributed to John Donne the 16th century poet:

> *God and the doctor we both alike adore,*
> *But only when in trouble, not before,*
> *The trouble o'er, both are alike requited,*
> *God is forgotten and the doctor slighted.*

I do not know the origin of the second epigram, but in the current age of high expectation and demand for immediate gratification, it is highly relevant:

> Be not the first by whom the new is tried,
> Nor yet the last, to cast the old aside.

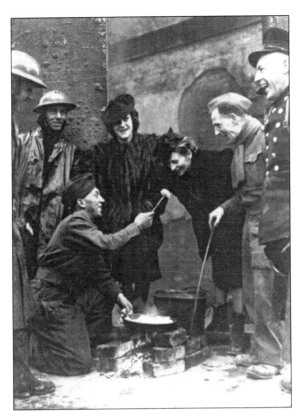

JC's mother, Millicent, during the Blitz 1941.

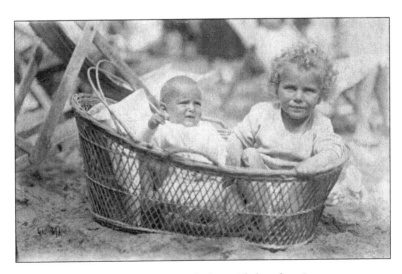

Starting Out - JC as a baby with brother Stuart.

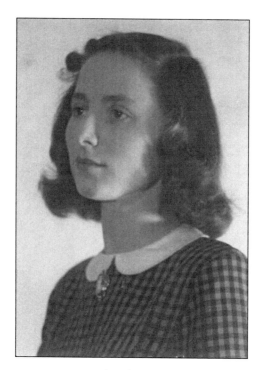

Pearl in her teens.

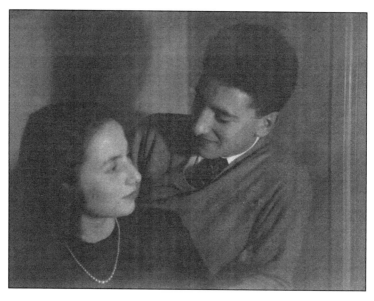

JC and PC - Young love, 1948.

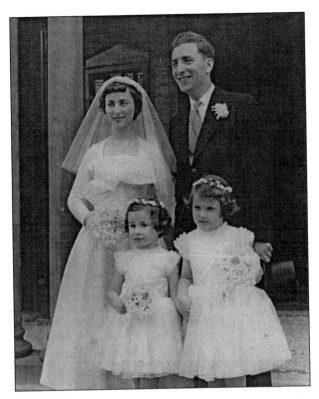

Wedding with bridesmaids Katherine and Stecia, 1952.

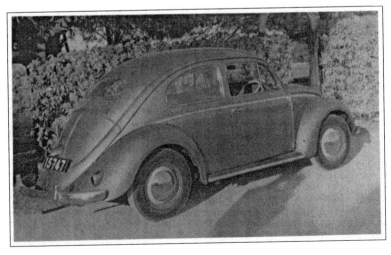

First car - Malta 1954.

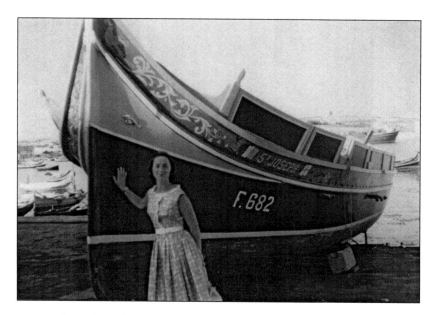

PC with Maltese fishing ship (Luzzu). Note 'evil eye' above her head.

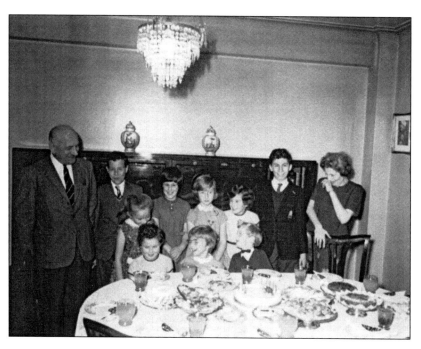

Debbie's 3rd birthday party with cousins and JC's parents, 1960.

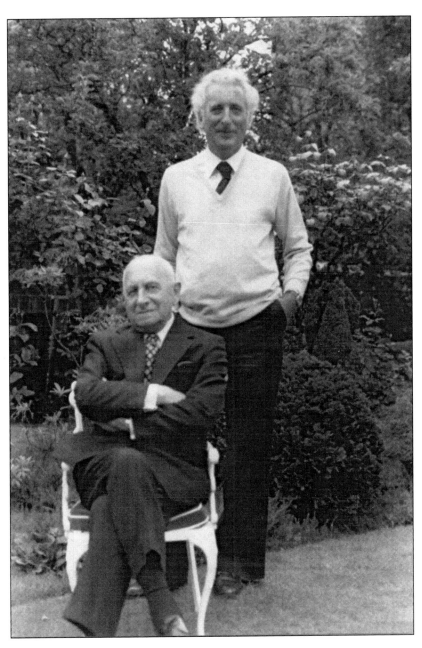

JC entering middle age with father, Bernard, 1972.

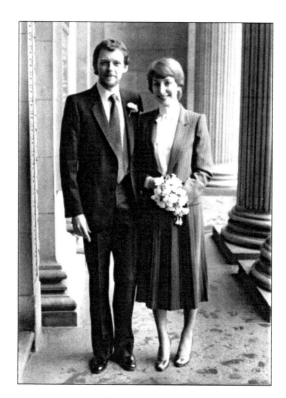

Marriage of Joanna and John, 1980.

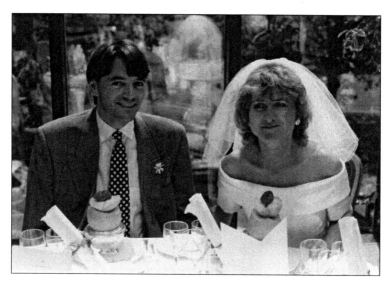

Marriage of Debbie and Steven, 1991.

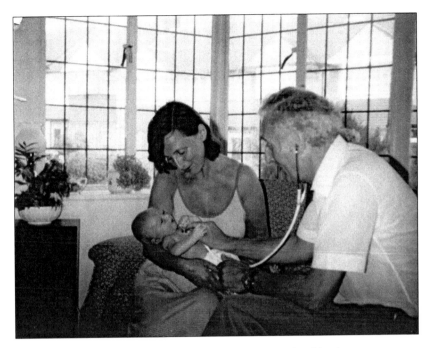

First grandchild, Tom, 1982. 'Just checking'.

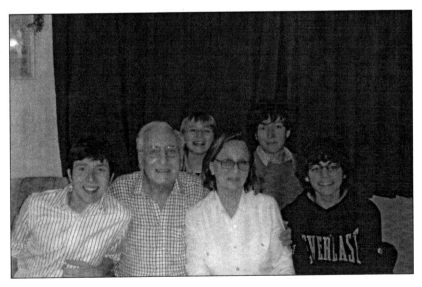

JC and PC with young grandsons.

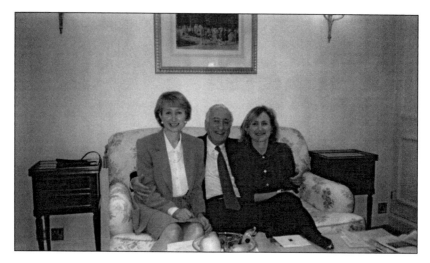

JC, proud father of Jo and Debbie.

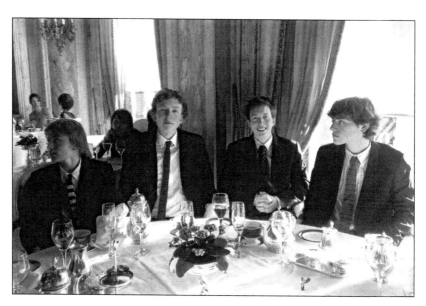

Grandsons Ollie, Tom, Matt and Alex dining at the Ritz, 2007.

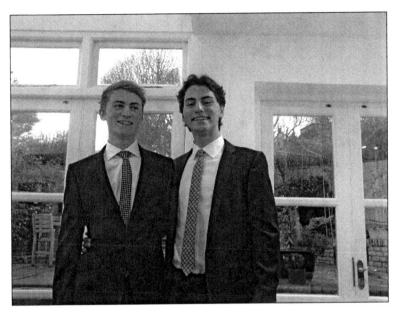

Grandsons Alex and Ollie starting out in the world, 2011.

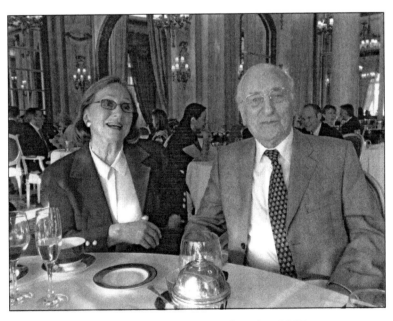

JC and PC dining out at the Ritz, 2007.

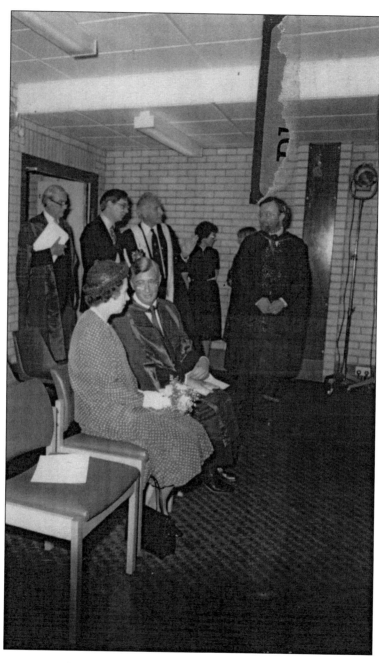

JC and members of the Department of General Practice,
St. Bartholomew's Hospital, with the Queen and
Duke of Gloucester, 1980s.

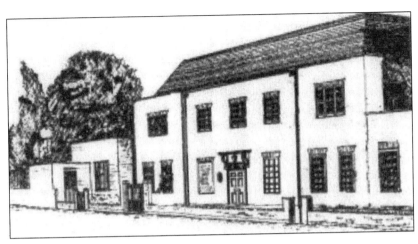

Sketch of Stamford Hill Group Practice.

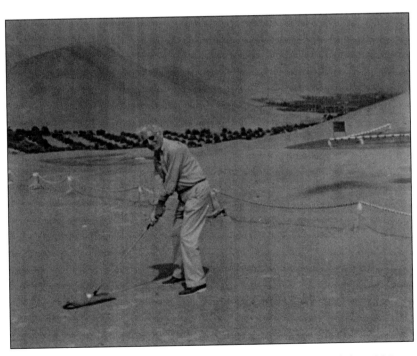

Golf on world's largest bunker, where it never rains - Chile, 1995.

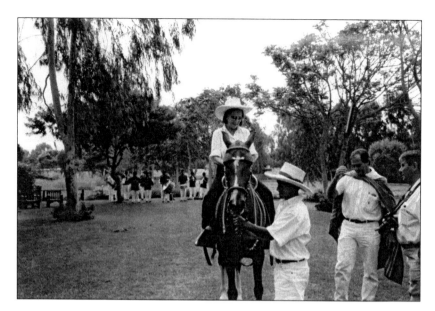

PC and 'friend' - Peru, 1994.

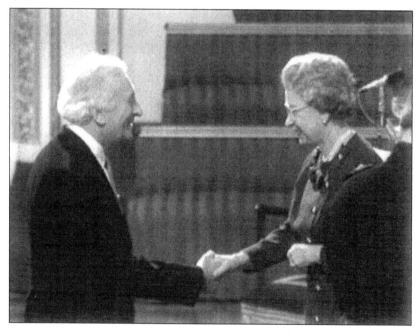

Receiving the MBE, 1992.

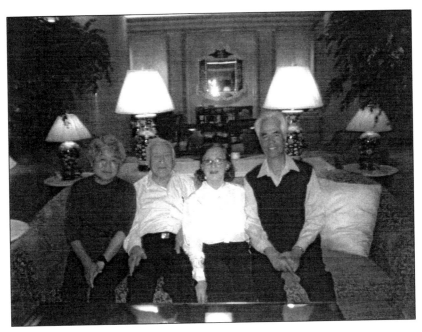

Together with our Chinese cousins - Beijing, 2008.

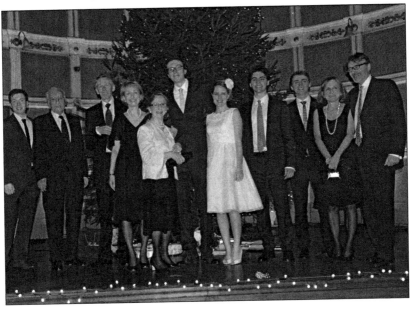

Family at Tom and Sophie's wedding, 2011.

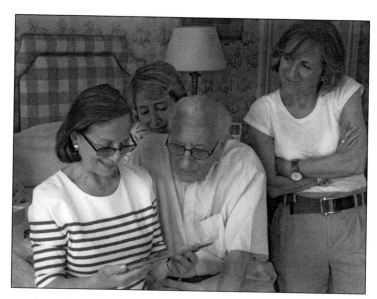

JC and PC celebrating their Diamond Wedding with Jo
and Debbie, 2012.

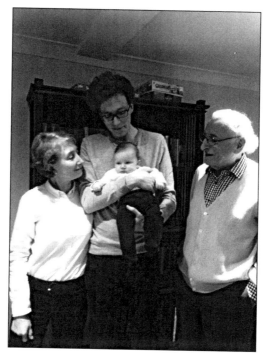

Four Generations, December 2013

CHAPTER XIV

Sweet and Sour

My intention in this chapter is to write about some of my memories from the early days of practice. As a GP sees "all of life passing" during a whole career, I thought I would mix some experiences that left me happy or amused ("sweet"), with others that left me drained or even temporarily depressed ("sour"). I am aware that the title brings to mind more an order given in a Chinese restaurant than experienced in the surgery, so I will add a category to the above in order that I can introduce an anecdote under the heading "I wish I could have said that" but was constrained through politeness or perhaps to avoid embarrassing or upsetting anyone. Names and identities have, of course, been changed and in some cases the narrative has been slightly altered to protect the confidentiality of those concerned, and maybe to spice up the story just a little.

A young Chinese lady who had recently registered with the practice, but I had not met before, came to see me with a much older man who turned out to be her grandfather. He had arrived in the UK on holiday a few days earlier and, like most new arrivals, had been informed of the wonderful benefits of our "free" health service, and in particular the even greater benefit that was available at the world-renowned Moorfields Eye Hospital for his rapidly failing vision. He spoke no English, his granddaughter very little, but after some time it became clear that he was requesting a letter to attend Moorfields while he was here on holiday, for treatment of his near blindness. It took even longer to explain that this was not possible under the regulations, and they left, I suspect to trail round other GPs with a view to finding one more accommodating to their wishes. It was only after they had gone (and I never saw them again), that it occurred to me that it might have been easier just to give him a letter addressed to the hospital stating, "This is to introduce Mr. ... who complains of numbers 21, 43, and 13."

On a more sombre note, I recall the adorable face of a six-year-old child, trustingly clutching his mother's hand and carrying out every instruction to "open his mouth", "say 99" and anything else I asked him to do. None of us knew at that moment that within 24 hours he would be dead, having been viciously attacked and beaten by a crazed tenant in the house in which he lived, and for no known motive whatsoever. The despair and distress of his mother is a memory I carry with me to this day. I also recall trying to comfort a mother, one of whose sons had climbed to the roof of their 10-storey council flat and thrown himself off. Even more difficult was trying to comfort her two years later when her other son did exactly the same thing.

On a "sweeter" topic, I recall two episodes that demonstrate in an amusing way the dangers that lurk when the normal lines of communication get crossed, which is not uncommon when language and nuances between people differ.

It was a long time ago - so long that it was before we had the luxury of receptionists and secretaries and had to carry out all the duties normally assigned to ancillary staff ourselves. It was also at a time when immigrants were being encouraged to enter the country to carry out some of the tasks the home-grown population were finding increasingly distasteful, bringing with them their customs, culture and general attitude to life. He was from the West Indies and came to register, all 6ft 6inches of him, having been in the country for some time but only recently feeling the need to seek medical advice. I started filling in the registration card. One of the first questions was, "What are your first names?" "William Ewart Gladstone" he replied. I had come to recognise the West Indian habit of naming their offspring after famous people, but these were usually cricketers or other sportsmen whose achievements made them feel proud. Naming them after long-dead politicians was new to me. I looked up at him from my chair, "What on earth do your friends call you?" I asked. "Oh, they just call me Tallboy," was his reply. Having completed the necessary form filling, I asked him what his problem was. He remained standing and said languidly, "It's my balls doc." Time was passing rapidly and I was aware of a full waiting room, so I concluded the quickest way to deal with the problem was to examine him and with this in mind, I asked him to drop his trousers, which he did equally as languidly, but with perhaps a touch of surprise. He had remained standing so I had to leave my chair and drop onto my knees to reach the correct height. I could see nothing obviously wrong, but felt keenly the incongruity of being on my knees and staring doggedly at his nether regions. Finally I was awakened from my soporific state by feeling rather than observing him looking down on the top of my head and asking, "What you doing, doc?" "Trying to see what is causing your pain," I replied. A look of complete disbelief came over him, "The balls of my feet, doc," he explained as if to a stupid child, but not one as stupid as I felt.

Some time later, a young Greek woman came to see me. By now we had a receptionist to do the paper work, but it soon became clear that the young woman's command of English was minuscule and mine of Greek non-existent. It took me twenty minutes to get her to understand my request that she should return the next day with a friend who could speak English. I was reassured that she understood the request by the large smile she gave me and as she left I heard her muttering to herself, "Tomorrow, friend, speak English". True to her word she returned the next day accompanied by a male friend who sat in the "patient's chair" and after the usual preliminary politeness I asked him to ask his companion what was her problem. "Oh, I don't speak Greek," he said in perfect English. After so many years have passed, I can no longer remember the outcome, but I certainly learnt the importance of making oneself clear and unambiguous when trying to be helpful.

I used to play tennis most Sunday mornings in Regent's Park. We were a regular foursome and one of the group took it upon himself to book the court. In the probably mistaken belief that it would add to his cache and gain him some benefits, he always booked it in my name, emphasising the word "doctor". As we arrived at the court, inevitably the man who took our money and had made the booking would greet him with a deferential tug of the hair and a bright, "Good morning, doctor". The rest of us just received a surly nod. One morning, on the next court were a couple of elderly gentleman who regularly played singles together but never once did I see them score points against each other (I later discovered that they were both psychiatrists and concluded that rivalry was frowned upon as being too dangerous for their comfort). On this particular morning, in the middle of their game, one of them slipped and fell flat on his face: he lay there with blood streaming down from a very large gash across the middle of his face. As the eyes of the other three in our game looked upon me as the natural saviour of a very unpleasant situation, I stood my ground, looked coolly at my partner (the one who always did the booking) and said, "After you, doctor". The look of disgust on the face of the booking clerk, as he discovered that his "favourite doctor" failed to act in an emergency, was only surpassed by my friend's intense embarrassment as he tried to explain that he wasn't a doctor after all. Unfortunately I could not enjoy the moment as much as I would have liked, as I had to leave the game to attend to the injured party.

Mavis and Margaret were two charming sisters who lived together, but were the only two remaining members of their family and still struggled to cope with living in the old family home, which was a very large Victorian house on three floors. They were respectively 96 and 92 years of age, and both very deaf. They were on my routine visiting list and I tried to see them at least once a month (it was accepted that the GP acted as doctor, nurse, social worker and companion and these routine visits were highly regarded by the patients, but in terms of "evidence-based medicine" they sometimes achieved very little other than a social advantage.) In the early 1980s it became possible to directly employ practice nurses, but in those early days, we did not really appreciate how best to deploy them within the practice team. District nurses provided a service of varying quality for the patients' medical needs, such as injections, bathing, dressings and bowel disturbances. Some extended this service for no other reason than they were genuinely kind and caring people, while others, alas, rushed in and out of the homes with very little in the way of empathy. As we did not actually employ them, they worked to their own rules and consequently, although we worked in full co-operation with some of them, we never saw or heard from others (I was called once to a diabetic lady in a coma, and it emerged that the district nurse had visited daily for the previous month, but on receiving no reply to her single ring on the bell, went on to the next client and never reported her failure to gain entrance to anyone).

To return to my story: we had employed a young, pretty and very efficient nurse, and I felt it would be a good idea if she took over some of the routine home visits. To initiate the process, I suggested she should come with me to introduce herself to the old sisters and to discuss what benefit she might be able to add to their care. Unfortunately I had forgotten to let the sisters know we were visiting at a different time from usual. The front door of the house was approached from the road up about ten steps, and having negotiated these steps, I rang the bell, and remembering their deafness, knocked as loudly as I could on the door. It was in vain, and after a further three attempts we were about to leave, when a window from a house across the road was opened, and a woman's head appeared and shouted across to us, "They are very deaf you know. Perhaps they can't hear you." Yes I did know, but realising I had been recognised, leaving without entering would look very uncaring. So I shouted back to her, "Would you mind phoning them and telling them we are here, so that they can open the door." (No mobile phones to help us on our way in 1980.) Agreeing this was a good idea, she went back into her house to make the call. By this time ten minutes had elapsed: I had many other calls to make and I was beginning to regret my plan to introduce the nurse on that particular day. A further few minutes passed, during which I continued to try and make myself heard on the doorbell and knocker. And then two things happened in rapid succession. I heard through the door the "thump, thump" of elderly arthritic feet slowly descending the stairs to answer the front door bell, and then the ring of the telephone within the house as our good Samaritan finally got through on her phone. To my horror, the "thump, thump" of approaching feet changed to "umph, umph" of retreating feet up the stairs, and I heard the voice of Margaret calling to me, "Just a minute, I have to answer the phone!" We could only respond to the Laurel and Hardy situation that we had created with a rueful laugh, and wait a further five minutes before we could finally enter the house.

While on the subject of home visits, another comes to mind. It was a Sunday morning and I was on call for the rota of doctors that we had organised in order to have some time free from the practice. The daughter of a patient who was unknown to me had called me. It was mid-winter and her mother was feeling very poorly with a high fever. When I arrived I was greeted by the daughter who turned out to be no more than 13 or 14 and whose first words were, "Please accept my father's apologies but he was working until very late last night [he was a taxi driver] and is trying to catch up on his sleep." No problem. She took me up to her mother's room where I was introduced to one of the fattest ladies I had ever seen. She appeared to completely take over the double bed in which she was sitting up, heavily sweating from her fever. As it was one of those illnesses quickly recognised as "there is a lot of it about", history taking took very little time. Wanting to be a good doctor and do the job properly, I felt it necessary to examine her before pronouncing a diagnosis. With this in mind I reached for the bed covers and swept them right back in preparation for the examination. To my surprise, I then espied for the first time her husband who was no more that 5ft tall and very thin: he was lying at her side, fast asleep and completely obliterated by her gargantuan proportions. He was still sleeping as I more gently replaced the covers and toned my voice down so as not to disturb him. As part of the continuing examination, I bent down on one knee in order to palpate her abdomen. As I was doing this I was slowly becoming aware that my right knee was getting wetter and wetter. I looked down, only to find I had inadvertently put my flexed knee into the chamber pot under the bed, which as you have probably guessed, was still full from the previous night. A whole new meaning for the expression "taking the piss!"

The words "heart sink" to describe a patient will be recognised by all doctors. The instant they enter the room, one's heart sinks. In the USA they are known as "gomers", an acronym for "get out of my examination room". Mavis was an embryo heart sink patient; only 27 years old but she had all the developing genes of a classical "heart sink". Talking of heart sink patients, an observation I made over the years was that all GPs had experience of them, but careful analysis showed that there was a limit to the number you could actually put up with at any one time. Somehow, once the limit was reached some mechanism came into play that blocked the recognition of other potential candidates. I do not know what became of them, but on discussing the phenomenon with other GPs we all agreed that when a heart sink patient left the practice for whatever reason, there was always another one on the waiting list to take their place!

To return to Mavis. She was rather bird-like with a voice that grated, and a rather unpleasant estuary accent: if you can imagine a female Ken Livingstone you will get the picture. She rarely had time for the niceties of a "Good morning," or "How are you today, doctor," but as usual came straight out with her reason for attending. "I hope it's all right, doctor, but I've got two complaints today." (This is known as the "double heart sink gambit".) "Well let's deal with one at a time," I said warily (perhaps I was hoping that after we had dealt with one problem she might have forgotten the other). "It's my periods," she whined, "I can't stand them. They are painful and heavy, with large clots and my stomach becomes all bloated. I lose my appetite and get very irritable, and the migraine I get with them is hardly bearable." This was going to take time! Perhaps encouraging her to tell me about her second complaint might help her to forget this one. "And what's your other complaint?" I asked tentatively. "Oh," she said, "I only get them once every three months!"

Paddy was not a patient of mine, but might well have been. He was actually our postman at home and had been so for many years (those were the days that postmen actually delivered the correct letters to the correct address and then put them through your post-box even if you lived on the top floor and there was no lift). It was not unusual for him to ring the bell and impart to me the latest district gossip, or if he felt he could get away with it, would slip in a medical problem of his own in the hope that he could have an "off the cuff" consultation. One day he rang the bell and when I answered he immediately apologised to me that he had been unable to deliver the post for the past fortnight as he had been ill. I must admit I had not really noticed his absence, but I enjoyed his company, so I asked what had been wrong with him. "It was my false teeth that were to blame." Feeling safe in the knowledge that as it was a dental problem I could be excused if I did not attempt to solve his problem, I asked him how had that stopped him working. "Well, you see I was carrying the sack of letters and gave this enormous sneeze." (Perhaps not so dental after all.) "How did that affect your teeth?" I asked. "Well, as I sneezed my teeth flew out of my mouth." I was getting just a little frustrated as to where this story was going. "Why did that stop you working for two weeks?" I asked. "Well as I bent down to pick them up, I got this terrible pain in my back and could not straighten up. It took two weeks in bed before the doctor said I could return to work." On another occasion, the post was very late, and just as I was beginning to despair of it coming at all, there was a welcome ring at the bell. Standing there, with a big grin on his face, but empty-handed, was my friend Paddy. "I've just called to tell you I forgot to take my bag of post out with me this morning." Instead of returning to pick up the sack, he had, apparently, gone round to all his "regulars" to apologise in person for his failure to deliver their post!

CHAPTER XV

Mostly Happy Times

At the time of writing, I have been involved in the medical field for over 60 years, six years as a student and junior doctor in hospital, three years in the RAF, 42 years as a general practitioner and so far 15 years retired but still involved, part time, in medical matters. Of the years in general practice, 41 were spent in Inner City Hackney at Stamford Hill. Rather than finding that my work environment had an adverse effect on my standard of practice, I found it uplifting. I also made sure that I maintained an interest in other aspects of medicine such as teaching and medical politics, while at the same time continuing to take time to follow my other interests of theatre, music, reading and sports.

Over the years I found myself associating with others whose purpose was to try and raise the standards of inner-city practice, and I believe that to a large extent we succeeded. By the time I retired, some of the best practices in the country, including two academic departments, were situated in our area and the immediate neighbouring area. I feel privileged to have been partly instrumental in setting up, together with four other colleagues, the Academic Department of General Practice at St Bartholomew's Hospital, which later amalgamated with the Royal London Hospital at Queen Mary College. I held the position of part-time senior lecturer for several years, during which time I met and worked with some of the most innovative and interesting people working in primary care.

The time spent teaching undergraduates was an eye-opening experience. I still remember, with some embarrassment, trying to teach the first group of clinical students at St Bartholomew's that were assigned specifically to learn about general practice. They were within a few months of qualifying (that period we have all gone through, when we think we have learnt all we need to know for the purpose of passing the final exams, and anything else is irrelevant, especially general practice, which everyone knew was what one practiced when you fell off the consultant ladder). As GPs ourselves, we were looked down upon by them and I have no doubt many of them in that group are now distinguished consultants in their chosen fields, but we very quickly recognised that they still had a lot to learn about people and their response to disease. The sessions (and there is no other way to describe the events that took place) developed in to a skirmish. By the end of the month the scores were just about equal – perhaps they won on penalties.

To paraphrase George Orwell, "all patients are equally interesting, but some are more equally interesting than others". An important part of learning medicine was the traditional method of "clerking" a patient while a student, which meant learning as much as you could from a patient to whom you had been assigned, by sitting at the bedside from the time they were admitted to their time of discharge. In those days this could be anything from a week to one or two months (day cases and rapid turnover were not even considered). From the point of view of relating with a patient, this was a definite advantage, especially to us students; I believe it also made the profession of nursing very much more a vocation than it is now. I am unsure whether the financial benefits gained from the present hospital philosophy of as near 100% occupancy rate as possible coupled with rapid discharge are really as positive as we are led to believe.

One patient I found myself clerking was a bright, middle-aged single lady with whom I had many interesting discussions on various topics while carrying out the duties a medical student had to perform. It transpired that she was the niece of a highly distinguished physician of a past age, who was recognised as the man who had developed the care of children into a specialty in its own right (he was known as "the father of paediatrics"). He had been knighted for his contributions and service to medicine and, along with other great teachers of the London Hospital (it only became Royal much later), his name was mentioned with awe around the hospital corridors. She confided in me that as a child she had been a fairly frequent visitor to his home in Harley Street and had come to the conclusion that he must have disliked children very much as they had to be "seen and not heard". They even had to take their shoes off within his home to reduce the noise they made. Hearing this, it became easier to believe the rumour that was prevalent in the hospital, that one of the contemporary paediatricians became so angry if a child cried on his ward round that the nurses had taken to giving them all a dose of chloral (a sedative in fairly common use) before he appeared. Looking back, I think the veracity of this is highly doubtful, a view I came to when I tasted chloral some years later: it is absolutely foul.

I blush with shame when I recall another habit prevalent in the casualty (now accident and emergency) department. Being in the heart of the East End, many of the clients were what we looked upon as down-and-outs. Some had discovered that if they could convince the "doctor" on duty (not infrequently a nurse or student) that they were truly unwell, they could spend the night on one of the comfortable trolleys in the cubicles, or if they were really lucky, spend a night or two in the wards. Not surprisingly, some overplayed their hand and having been successful on one occasion would try and repeat the performance. The rapid change in student personnel made recognition of the persistent offenders difficult (although some of the ex-service students were pretty adept at recognising them). Accordingly, a black book was kept of those poor souls who were deemed "unfit to be unfit". If they were recognised, they were allowed a finite time to tell their story, and then irrespective of whether they were in need or not, they were prescribed the "powerful cure-everything" medicine which we knew as *mist asafetida* or, in the vernacular, and for good reason, *mist diabolica*. It was composed of a mixture of harmless but the foulest smelling and tasting ingredients to be found in the pharmacopoeia. They rarely came back.

One patient remains as a painful memory to this day. He was the first real patient with whom I identified strongly. There were many more to come, but like one's first love, the memory lasts. My first job after qualifying was in the orthopaedic department. Peter (not his real name) was a year or two younger than me, but like me had just graduated from university. To celebrate the occasion he and some friends went down to Southend (or some similar coastal resort) where they went bathing in the sea. Under the influence of the sun, beer and the euphoria of having passed their exams, they looked for some adventure more exciting than straightforward bathing. They found what they were looking for in the shape of some moored fishing boats, one of which had a diving board attached to it. He accepted a bet to dive off the board into the sea, but tragically had not considered the influence of a receding tide, which had left the depth of the water much too shallow for such an attempt. His neck was broken, leaving him quadriplegic. No movement remained in his arms or legs and he had no bladder or bowel control. It was in this state that he was admitted into the hospital and in which I found him. For the next two months or so, I had daily contact with him and found it very difficult not to imagine myself in his position. I do not know what the final outcome was for Peter. The memory stays with me with great sadness, though, for such a wasted life.

One of the things about general practice is the interest experienced from the great variety of people one comes across. Some are interesting in a positive way, but others invoked the necessity of trying to remember the motto of the London Hospital Medical College, namely *homo sum humani nihil a me alienum puto*. Roughly translated this means *I am a man and there is nothing about humans that is alien to me*. Many is the time when having to carry out an unpleasant examination or procedure I have had to remind myself of this. One such family were quite pleasant and we got on well together in spite of my awareness that they had a criminal streak. I was not so happy when the son, no doubt following the family tradition, was arrested and later found guilty of having tricked himself into the home of an elderly gentleman, tying him up and producing a knife, saying he had come "to sell him a life insurance policy". The deal was "either he paid him £5,000 or his life would be in serious jeopardy". Another young patient was convicted of rape, and I experienced strong mixed feelings in trying to help his mother come to terms with what her son had done (or, as she was convinced, had not done). Another patient was convicted of a crime serious enough to have him sent to the notorious prison at Dartmoor. He, too, I had found to be a congenial character in his home life, and we had had several discussions before his downfall. It must also have had some effect on him, since he appears to have spoken highly of his doctor in Civvy Street to other inmates in the prison. As a result I found myself being sought after by at least two ex-convicts after their release from Dartmoor, seeking medical advice. All I can say is that they were very pleasant people and I found some difficulty in reconciling what my conscience told me I should have thought of them when experience told me the opposite.

Another patient I knew owned and edited a soft porn magazine. After I had visited him at home a couple of times I became aware that some of his "copy" was obtained by photographing the models in his own home. One evening I was called to see him as he had quite a severe chest infection. (He was a very heavy smoker and was later to die of the lung cancer his habit had caused.) It transpired that, although he was ill enough to request a visit, he was not too ill to continue working. The door was opened, to my surprise, by a nun. Not the type of nun to be found in the musical *The Sound of Music*, but a young, attractive young woman about whom it was not too difficult to imagine a nubile figure under her convent attire. She pointed me into the front room, used by my patient as his bedroom, and disappeared into the next-door room, emanating from which I noticed a bright light. The penny dropped soon after I started taking a history of the illness, as each question I asked was punctuated by a *slap, slap* sound followed by "Ouch,

ouch!" It was coming from the next room. My patient apologised for the distraction, explaining that they were in the middle of photographing a sado-masochistic scene for the next issue of his magazine. As they were being paid by the half hour, it would be too expensive to stop just because I was there . . .

There was one occasion when he arrived at surgery rather out of breath having hurried up the hill from his home to my surgery. Unlike him (his consultations were usually of some significance) he brought up a minor problem, which was very quickly disposed of, and then said, "I have really come to ask you a favour." I was all ears: after all, this was quite a distraction. I was rather surprised at the nature of his request. "We are in the middle of filming and we desperately need a stethoscope: can I borrow yours for an hour or two?" True to his word, the stethoscope was returned via taxi within the hour, but I still have vivid fantasies as to what purpose my stethoscope might have been used. Discretion being the better part of valour, I gave it a good wash before using it again.

Another patient, let us call him Charles, had been previously married, and had grown up children. On one occasion he introduced me to his new and very young wife, who herself had a very young child. At first all seemed to go well, but after a couple of years of marriage I was visited by his grown up daughter who was very worried at the deterioration in her father's health. I was disbelieving when she expressed her fear (by now, in her mind, a certainty) that her father was being poisoned by his new wife in order that she might benefit from his will. He was, in fact, being prescribed tablets for a weak heart, and when I reluctantly investigated her claim, I found that the quantities of tablets that had been prescribed did not match the amount he was meant to take. I advised taking the tablets away, much to the fury of his wife, but to the great improvement in health of Charles. He refused to report the matter to the police, but in any case, by this time his wife had packed all her belongings (and some of his) and done a bunk, never to be seen again.

A memorable patient I encountered was not my patient at all. I was in Switzerland – the reason why I should be visiting a Swiss hospital at all escapes me, but I think it was out of interest to see how other systems worked, while I was there on holiday. I met a three-year-old child lying in a hospital bed, the poor girl encased in plaster-of-paris covering both arms and at least one leg. The history was that she had accidentally fallen off a table while playing around at home. At the time we had, in this country, become aware of the work from America concerning the so-called battered baby syndrome. Seeing this child, the possibility that this was a case of non-accidental injury was high on my priority list. I suggested to the Sister in charge of the ward, acting as our guide, this possibility. She was of the old school, the like of whom we have not seen for many years, and I felt intimidated when she fixed me with a glare from her dark brown eyes and said, "I have heard of such things happening, but in Switzerland people do not do such wicked things!" I wonder how long it took them to find out that they might.

This next paragraph might be subtitled "Near Virgin Births". Four young women I have encountered over the years have remained in memory. The first was a young girl of sixteen to whom I had been called at 10 o'clock at night because her mother thought she might have appendicitis. "Her stomach pains were bad." She was previously unknown to me, but when I arrived she was lying in her mother's double bed, whimpering but otherwise looking flushed but well. There was no fever or raised pulse rate and her tongue was clean. The history had revealed she had been having the pains over the past two hours. It was not difficult to observe, when the bedclothes were pulled back, that she was in the last stages of pregnancy and the early stages of labour, but her mother was completely unaware of this possibility and apparently blind to the bulging abdomen. I felt that fairly urgent action was called for and realising that this would be best achieved without mother being present, at least for the time being, I asked her if she could bring in some water that had been boiled in the kettle so that I could carry out a "special test" (I had no idea to what test I was referring). With mother out of the room I immediately confronted the girl and asked if she had any idea that she was not only pregnant, but labour had probably started. The confrontational approach proved effective, as she admitted to the possibility but in no way was her mother to know. In the circumstances, dealing with the situation without mother knowing was not a possibility and I pointed this out to her. When mother returned with the water (which was quickly forgotten) I informed her of the situation, at which point she turned to her daughter and said, "But you have never been out with a boy!" By this time the daughter had realised that nothing but complete honesty was going to resolve the situation, and she replied tearfully, "I did once, last spring, when I told you I was going out for a bike ride." I left unstated the thought running through my mind. "I wonder if it was one of those bikes with a crossbar!"

One morning whilst shaving, a phone call was received and relayed to me by my wife: the message said no more than "Gillian (I've changed the name) had belly ache and would I please visit her urgently as she had to go to school." On an urgency scale of one to ten this was not very high, so I finished shaving, had my breakfast and visited on my way to surgery. The home was a well-kept council flat and the family a middle class Jewish one. It did not take long for me to ascertain that Gillian was in the later stages of labour, and could be expected to deliver at any moment. A 999 call very quickly secured a blue light ambulance. Gillian disappeared into hospital and had her baby safely, but it was some time later that I learned that arrangements had been made to have the baby taken away for adoption before poor Gillian was even allowed to see it. Notwithstanding the trauma, and ignorant, as most of us were then, of post-traumatic stress syndrome and the need for therapy, Gillian was quickly back to her normal life and continuing at school. Almost exactly two years later, again while shaving, another phone message was received by my wife from Gillian's mother, asking me to visit as soon as possible as Gillian had a recurrence of her "tummy trouble". This time I finished shaving in record time, dressed over my pyjamas and left without breakfast, arriving at Gillian's within 20 minutes of the call.

Unlikely as it would appear, she was again in the later stages of labour, the ambulance had to be called and the baby snatched away for adoption before Gillian could see it. I am still amazed that not only did Gillian return to an apparently normal life, but continued to consult me for several years even after she had become married and moved out of the district, and had started a family of her own. This one she had kept.

My third case is, perhaps, the strangest of all three. Giselle was 23-years-old and her family were orthodox Jewish from Morocco. Both her religious and ethnic background made sex before marriage a taboo subject. By the time she first found the courage to consult me she was already at least 16 weeks pregnant. She could not understand why her belly was expanding. After abdominal examination had confirmed that pregnancy was the most likely diagnosis, she was genuinely surprised as she assured me she had "never had sex with a boy". Careful probing eventually disclosed that she did admit to kissing and cuddling and what we used to innocently call petting. She assured me she had never removed all her clothes. Referral, under the strictest secrecy (she correctly assumed she would have been banished from her home if her parents found out), to a gynaecologist confirmed that she was pregnant, but her circumstances were such that her mental condition would be severely affected if the pregnancy was allowed to continue, and that termination was justified on medical grounds. The gynaecologist also confirmed her story in as much as he found that she was still virgo-intacta, thus proving that in a highly fertile couple, heavy petting can lead to a viable pregnancy. As she was so far advanced in pregnancy, intravaginal termination was unsuitable, and she had to undergo a hysterotomy – termination by what, in reality, is equivalent to a caesarean section of a normal birth. Honour and her own safety were saved, but only temporarily: two years later she consulted me again with exactly the same problem. Once again she was 14 to 16 weeks pregnant, but still denied absolutely that she had "made love". Referral to the same gynaecologist was necessary, and I was not too surprised when he sent me a letter stating, "that for the first time in my career, I have had to perform two terminations on the same patient who still remains a virgin!"

The fourth case has a rather different denouement. Ruth was only 14 and was dragged in by her mother because of her discovery of a large abdominal swelling, equal to a near-term pregnancy. Her tearful daughter admitted she had had fairly regular sexual intercourse with her 15-year-old boyfriend and from her point of view she was happy to keep the baby and marry the father. Not, perhaps, a very practical solution. Examination appeared to confirm the presence of a pregnancy of about 30 weeks' duration, but I could not hear the heart, and she said she could feel no movement. At the time I was a clinical assistant in the gynaecological outpatient department of our local hospital and it was not difficult to arrange for her to be seen by the consultant at the next clinic. His more expert examination revealed that she might not be pregnant at all, but he thought she might have a large ovarian cyst. Very unusual, but possible, and an examination under anaesthesia (EUA) was quickly arranged, the girl and her mother having been warned that operation might be necessary if the EUA showed that it was indeed a cyst that was causing the swelling. As the case was so interesting I arranged to be present at the procedure, and sure enough a giant-sized ovarian cyst was confirmed; operation for its removal followed immediately. At operation, the news was not good. The cyst had destroyed most of the ovary and due to its position and size the whole right ovary had to be removed. In addition, the left ovary also had a cyst, somewhat smaller, but there was an obvious risk that the same that had happened on the right might have occurred on the left. A decision had to be made whether to remove her left ovary, with obvious dire consequences, or risk leaving well alone. After some deliberation, the latter course of action was followed, but she was told that her chances of future pregnancies were very small. As the years passed, she did marry the boyfriend and had two normal children of her own. The whole episode when she was only 14-years-old was happily forgotten; although unfortunately the marriage did not survive her husband's bad behaviour towards her.

CHAPTER XVI

Balint and Balintism

I have previously spoken about the influence Michael Balint and his teaching had on my professional life, and also, it must be said, to my greater understanding of all aspects of human behaviour, whether as patients or acquaintances. In a 2008 article in the *British Medical Journal* (*BMJ*), Jeremy Holmes posed the question: "Are we all Balintians now?" In the sense that Balint's teaching still influences the way we practice and think as general practitioners, I believe the answer must be yes; but in an era of evidence-based medicine, it is no longer so fashionable to admit to it.

Michael Balint was Hungarian by birth and while still practicing there worked with some of the giants of Freudian psychoanalysis. Driven out by the political situation and racial intolerance of the 1930s, he came to England and worked as a psychoanalyst, eventually achieving an honorary consultancy at the Tavistock Clinic (now a large building at the bottom of Fitzjohns Avenue, but previously a fairly small house in Beaumont Street, in the Harley Street area of the West End). His interest and research into the doctor patient relationship, shared by his second wife Enid a lay analyst, was the unrecognised effect that the interaction between a doctor and his patient had on the outcome of a disease. It was also Balint's intention to see whether a greater understanding of the role that the doctor played in the transaction would help GPs understand and cope better with the difficult problems they encountered. This was the early 1950s and the NHS was only three years old. Those of us who were in practice at that time were well aware that a free health service had increased the demand on services enormously. The prediction of the Beveridge report – namely, that as people became eligible for medical care previously denied them because of financial poverty the need for treatment would lessen – had proved to be a false hope: disorders previously tolerated were now coming to light as people realised they could seek expert care. As the doctors of first contact, GPs were finding that the pressure put upon them threatened to overwhelm them (and almost did).

GPs in the front line of this battle reacted in various ways. Many merely abdicated their responsibility and did no more than write a prescription, give a certificate of unfitness to work on request, or give a note to the local hospital asking for a second opinion. Since time was at a premium and secretaries to type proper letters of referral were almost unknown, consultants tended to complain that many of the letters from GPs they received said little more than "please see and treat". (It was not long before I recognised that many of the letters coming back from the consultant said no more than "seen and treated", which was not very helpful.) General practice was in a state of chaos and as a consequence those of my generation had to make a conscious decision whether to join the trend and accept that a pen, prescription pad and book of certificates were all one needed, in the process foregoing all the ideals we once held while at medical school, or alternatively reject the NHS and emigrate to practice abroad. Fortunately there was one further option and that was to resolve to stay and practice medicine at as high a standard as one could achieve. To digress: it might be asked what standard could reasonably be expected of a GP practicing within a service that only allowed a few minutes per patient. When teaching trainees in general practice, I would try to convince them that one should always *aim* at 100% perfection. This would ensure that at least they could hope to achieve a 60% to 70% success rate towards their goal; if one accepted only 60% to 70% as the maximum achievable, it is likely that only 30% to 40% success would be reached.

Those of us sufficiently stimulated and energetic enough to attempt to practice a high standard of medicine looked around for ways of achieving this goal. There were probably other influences at work, but in my own case I found that there were two important developments that I found helpful and whose causes I espoused with enthusiasm. John Hunt (later Lord Hunt), together with other stalwarts, set up the College of General Practitioners, which gave stability, status and standards ("the three s's") to all aspiring GPs. This became so successful that over 60 years later, and now the Royal College of General Practitioners, it is recognised worldwide, with many other countries now having their own colleges devoted to general practice. The other important factor was Michael Balint and from the small group of GPs who had responded to an advertisement for doctors who were interested in the interaction between doctors and patients, worldwide groups have evolved. Regular seminars were held under the guidance of a psychoanalyst; the word "leader" was never used, even though Michael himself found it very difficult not to lead! In order to be accepted into a group one had to commit to at least two years involvement, which has probably proved too hard for the present generation of GPs to accept. As a consequence, in the UK at least, the number of flourishing Balint groups is minimal, although in some other countries they are still ongoing. Notwithstanding the decline of active groups, many of the discoveries that were made are now part of the fabric of present-day general practice.

In 1972 a working party was set up by the RCGP that produced a report in book form entitled *The Future General Practitioner*. The working party consisted of six prominent GPs of whom five had been attendees at Balint groups. I have no doubt in my mind that their views, as expressed in the report, were very Balint orientated and it is one of the reasons why the answer to the question posed at the beginning of this chapter must be a resounding yes.

From Balint's first group of GPs the book *The Doctor his Patient and the Illness* was born and the teaching of Balint became more widespread. (Note that the illness in the title stands alone and does not belong to either the doctor or the patient – an important distinction.) As the seminars became more widespread and the interest in the aims for what Balint stood grew, more publications arose from the research being carried out within the groups. Max Klein wrote *Absent* (a study of truancy). Aaron Lask produced *A Study of Night Calls* in which the feelings (both positive and negative) invoked in the doctor when called out at night were studied with much insight. Michael Courteney produced *Sexual Discord in Marriage*. *Virgin Wives* by Leonard Friedman was a study of non-consummation within marriage, and later titles include the one in which I was personally involved, *Six Minutes for the Patient*. This was written as a result of the work being carried out by the group when, sadly, Michael became ill and died. Enid, his wife, was co-leader of the group and we agreed to continue the research and the final work was published under the editorship of Enid Balint and Jack Norrell. It was fashionable then, in the 1970s, to complain that the time allowed for a consultation, an average of about six minutes, was not nearly long enough. If only we were allowed more time, we would be able to practice at a higher standard! What we set out to do, rather than moan about the situation, was to recognise the six minutes as a fact and ask what could be done within that time that would make us better doctors. I claim authorship of the title that we eventually chose. I remembered a novel of a few years previously called *Seven Minutes* in which the author, Irvine Wallace, states that he had named the novel after the research of the Kinseys, who had discovered that seven minutes was the average time it took a woman to reach orgasm during sexual intercourse. It seemed to me that on this basis six minutes would describe our objectives ideally. Other groups, working with the Balints, produced, among other titles, *The Doctor his Patient and the Group* and *Treatment or Diagnosis*.

When we commenced our research for *Six Minutes for the Patient* we were aware that very often at the end of a consultation the patient would hint at the real reason they had come, but had perhaps been too diffident, or afraid, to mention it beforehand.

The French would refer to this as the *esprit d'escallier* or "thought on the stairs". As we studied the contents of the consultation, and the significance of the interactions between doctor and patient, we noted that very often what the patient first said might also be of great significance, but was often ignored. Turning to chess for our inspiration, we used the term *opening gambit* to describe this phenomenon. On one occasion, when the discovery was fresh in my mind, I was asked if I would host a keen follower of Michael Balint from Germany who was spending a three-month sabbatical in England studying general practice and how it might be influenced by exposure to the Balints' training. At the end of what was to me a routine morning's surgery (but to him a first exposure to our national health service) we discussed the contents of the consultations. Inevitably the question arose of whether I had noted the significance of recognising an opening gambit in a routine morning surgery. I was amused when after a few minutes discussion he said with a heavy German accent, "Yes, I have always known the significance of the 'thought at the door', but you have demonstrated how the opening gambit may also contain significant information. But tell me, why do you, in this country, bother with the middle?"

My introduction to Michael Balint was through my brother-in-law who was a GP who had been introduced to the seminars and was attending one run by Michael at the Tavistock Clinic. As I have already described, jobs were hard to find when I came out of the RAF in 1956. I had eventually been accepted as a trainee in Paddington. The work was not too arduous and I wanted to use some of the spare time I had in filling in some of the gaps that were left due to my having to join the RAF after less than a year doing hospital jobs. I had been accepted by the Royal National Ear Nose and Throat Hospital for a useful training job in which they offered a once-a-week "sit in" training post for six months, and then a once-weekly clinical assistantship in the hospital for a further six months. As both posts were paid it also gave a useful boost to my very inadequate pay. I had also written to the Skin Hospital in Leicester Square asking if I could sit in on a weekly basis for three months with one of their consultants. I was invited to sit in with Dr. Mitchell-Heggs, a leading dermatologist, so two afternoons a week had been filled. (In those days morning surgeries finished at about 11am, then home visits were done and the afternoons were free until evening surgery commenced at 6 or 6.30pm. This allowed time to do postgraduate work if one was so inclined, but it did make for a long, hard day.)

Rather surprisingly, when I expressed interest in finding out more about the work of Michael Balint, my request to attend as an observer to the group in which my brother-in-law was a member was accepted, the only proviso being that I attend two seminars. (Later, Michael discouraged observers and made it the rule that you had to live a fair distance outside of London, otherwise you had to apply to be a full member. This, in turn, committed you to at least two years within a group.) I have always enjoyed group discussion and when I found that it was also a means by which I could express my doubts and shortcomings and share them with other like-minded GPs, I hastily applied for membership and was accepted into a group led by a colleague of Michael's at the Tavistock, Pierre Tourquet. He was a charming, thoughtful and very large man, soon, tragically, to be killed in a car accident while travelling on holiday in France. I remained a member of one group or another, under various leaders (I cannot think of another word to describe their function accurately) for the following 30 years. I believe I was a better doctor (or at least, more effective) for the experience, but others must judge me on that score. Being committed brought with it many responsibilities and much hard work. In the early years, if one was presenting a case it had to be from the current workload, and before meaningful discussion could take place you would be expected to know a fair amount about your patient. A basic rule was that clinical notes of the patient were not allowed but one had to report from memory. In this way the true feelings of the doctor could be displayed rather than a mere narration of boring facts. The expression "Who's got a case?" became the standard opening gambit of all Balint seminars. Often the presenting doctor would attempt to reduce the enormity of what he was about to communicate by introducing the case with the phrase, "This won't take very long..." Alas, as with patients who preface their consultation with "I won't keep you long, doctor" – or, even more ominously, "As you know, I never trouble you unless it is absolutely necessary" – this was rarely the case. The "long case" became the accepted norm. This did not refer to a grandfather clock, but to the fact that rather than a normal consultation, one had to bring back the patient by appointment (a true appointment system was a rarity in the 1950s and 1960s) for a protracted consultation, usually of about one hour's duration. This was usually at the end of evening surgery making that long day even longer.

History has recorded that the so-called permissive society occurred during the 1960s and early 70s. During this time I was heavily involved with Balint training and research, and I believe this helped me to adjust and accept what was an explosive change of attitude towards sexual mores. Especially as a doctor, one had to learn to accept changing behaviour patterns in one's patients and not to be seen as too paternalistic or forbidding. At the same time, our two daughters were in their teens and having to make their own adjustments. In 1969 or 1970 I was rather shocked to hear one of my colleagues state that, if he had a daughter who was still a virgin at the age of 18, he would be very worried for her. A year or two later I had to admit to mixed feelings when my own daughter asked my advice about starting on the contraceptive pill: proud that she felt she could ask, but somewhat regretful that my attitude towards sexual freedom was finally being dragged out of the middle ages.

There were some downside consequences of being a follower of Balint. Some GPs had found the psychiatric side of their practice to which they had become exposed so attractive that they left general practice for good and trained to become psychiatrists or psychotherapists. Balint always maintained that when this happened he had failed in his task of improving and understanding general practice. Unfortunately there also appeared to be a higher than average rate of broken marriages among the colleagues with whom I was associated. Whether this was because of the sexually accepted mores and experimentation of the 1960s or the negative influence of working with Balint I cannot say. No doubt self-awareness that was heightened by contact with Balint groups (he used to say that within two years of joining a group the doctor experienced a definite change of personality) played its part, but sadly several partnerships that appeared to be long lasting broke up over the time I knew them.

Before he died, a group of us were instrumental in forming the Society of Balint Medical Groups – apparently it was not acceptable to name a society after a living person – but soon after he died it was unanimously agreed that the name should be changed to the Balint Society, and it remains so to this day, even though the days of annual conferences and numerous working groups are over. I was honoured and privileged to be made president of the society in the 1980s.

In the early days there were several lady doctors attending the groups. Although working as GPs, a fair number were not full-time, and it was also the custom for much of the family-planning work to be carried out by females, presumably because contraception was considered to be predominantly a female problem. Recognising that the cases they were bringing to the seminars were not always relevant to the full time GPs present (and vice versa), they formed a break off group under the guidance of Tom Main, a psychoanalyst at the Cassel Hospital, which came to be known as (and still is) the Institute of Psychosexual Medicine. I also had the honour of being invited to be one of three honorary vice-presidents they appointed.

I could go on much longer on the subject of Balint, but before signing off, I will relate one anecdote that I will always associate with his name. It concerns a patient of mine. She was a very sexually attractive young woman, but of a very self-destructive personality, these powers often extending to those around her. She had reached the height of notoriety – written about in national newspapers – a few years earlier, when she had climbed on to the roof of one of London's large teaching hospitals, refusing to come down until her demands were met. (I'm afraid I no longer remember what these demands were.) As a young man, Michael had served in the Hungarian Army, and often quoted what he told us was the term used then for anyone suffering from backache. Whatever the cause the sufferer was always referred to as having "fucker's back", thus recognising the term might relate to being a "lazy f...er", a "sexy f...er" or any other sort of "f...er" How do these two facts marry up? I will call her Mary and she crawled in to see me almost on all fours, complaining of a terrible backache, describing how it had been much worse the previous evening but was now easing off. As I looked at her, with her make-up smeared and her hair hardly combed, but wearing a cocktail dress reaching only halfway down her thighs, I wondered what on earth had happened. As she sat down, the tip of a suspender attached to her stocking top was just visible. My mind went back to Michael's aphorism as I asked her to tell me the full story. She related how the day before she had reached her lowest ebb, realising she didn't have enough money to live the life she yearned after. Although admittedly sexually promiscuous, she had never succumbed to selling her favours for a direct cash transaction, nor would she ever consider it. However, under the influence of a friend's persuasion (and no doubt a little of the hard stuff) she had decided to give it a try, reassuring herself that it would be for once only. Having dressed for the occasion and making sure she looked her sexiest, she did what she had been informed was the best way to meet a client, namely go to a smart London hotel and sit in the foyer or lounge and wait for a suitable fish to snatch at the bait. With some trepidation she sat as instructed and was only slightly surprised that within a few minutes a smartly dressed foreign gentleman approached her. He looked clean and rich and appeared to her to be an ideal candidate, so she agreed to meet him in his room in ten minutes' time. When the ten minutes were up she decided to take the bull by the horns and go up to his room. As she went to rise, she found her back had completely locked and she could not get up from the chair. The outcome was that she spent the rest of the night in the armchair in the lounge of the hotel, but with her honour (as she judged it) intact. By the morning the pain had eased off enough to allow her to come and see me. I think you will agree that this was a classic case, in Balint's words, of a fucker's back.

CHAPTER XVII

Some of My Best Friends . . .

The subject of the orthodox Jewish community, who became a large part of my professional life over the 41 years I practiced in Stamford Hill, is uncomfortable because of the ambivalent feelings I have towards them. To explain, I must revisit my upbringing.

Religion has never been something for which I have had much time, but I respect the beliefs of all religions as long as they do not try and influence their fellow men to an undue extent. From a personal point of view, I am only two generations away from living the strictly orthodox life, my grandfather having been a leading orthodox Jewish figure in the East End of London and a supporter of the blossoming Lubavitch and Chabad factions in the early 20th century. He brought up his family in the same way that so many of my patients did: as strictly orthodox Jews, in a highly paternalistic society, in which father's word was only second to God's; and he maintained the right of being the interpreter of what God meant in his pronouncements. Of his four children, his only son died of typhoid, which he caught while visiting the family vineyards in what was then Palestine. This was just before I was born, so I did not know him, but I was named after him. Of his three daughters, my mother was the youngest and the rebel. Her two sisters both lived a religious life, one of whose family members remain highly religious through to the present generation. The other sister, and oldest of her family, had seven children with varying religious outcomes. I have spoken in another chapter of her only daughter, who died tragically young of tuberculosis just after the Second World War, leaving behind a Chinese dynasty. Of my aunt's six sons, they varied in their religious propensities from ultra-orthodox to converts to

Unitarianism. The descendants of my maternal grandparents' immediate family tended to remain religious. On the single occasion that I can remember a complete family get-together, which was about 20 years ago when my aunt celebrated her 100th birthday, the guests were truly a kaleidoscopic mixture of faiths and cultures. My father, on the other hand, was an only child with a very small extended family and although religious his family are much less complicated. The members can be counted on the fingers of both hands – well, perhaps adding the toes for the few more now forgotten by me.

As a child I remember recognising that orthodoxy in our home, if not exactly waxing and waning like the moon, at least ebbed and flowed like the tide. In some years Chanukah *gelt* (money) seemed to take precedence over Christmas presents, while in other years, and for no reason that I could fathom, Christmas seemed to be the dominant cause for celebration. Our Jewishness was never forgotten and we visited synagogue on a fairly regular basis, although Saturday services were often missed if there were more important things to do – or if my father's favourite football team were playing at home with an early kick-off. We attended synagogue in Egerton Road, later to become the road where our group practice was situated, and I recall how when it came to the time for the Rabbi to give his sermon there was a general exodus for the door until he had finished. I assumed, in my young mind, that this was so that one could go to the toilet, or perhaps have a smoke (didn't everyone in those days!) but gradually I realised that the true reason was much more prosaic. He was a bore and he went on far too long. On festivals, we went to a private synagogue run by family friends. The benefit of no sermons was offset by the disadvantage of the prolonged prayers, recited in their entirety, and the fact that everyone spoke only Yiddish.

Friday night was invariably family-supper night at home, and we would look forward to my father arriving home from work so that the ceremony could begin. (As I write this I must admit to a small doubt: my own anticipation of his presence was made happier because of the bars of chocolate he would bring home with him.) Traditional candles were always lit, but this was the responsibility of the distaff side of the family, so escaped my recognition of what was involved. Prayers before dinner – *Kiddush* over the wine, and blessing over the special plaited bread or *choler* – were made, and my brother and I, from a very early age, were made to say this prayer. Repetition led to familiarity and even now on the high holidays such as *Rosh Hashanah* (the Jewish new year) and *Yom Kippur* (the day of atonement) when my own family join us, my children and grandchildren believe that I have knowledge of Hebrew that allows me to read it straight from the book. In fact I am only repeating, as a reflex reaction, the words that I had been made to recite, parrot fashion, as a child.

On Saturdays I would wake up with trepidation: were we to be taken to synagogue, where I knew I was destined to be bored? Or was Clapton Orient playing at home with an early kick off? At the time we lived in Stamford Hill, home to so many middle-class Jews who had moved out of the East End in search of a better life. Whether it was coincidence or quirk I am not sure, but as I returned to the area and practiced as a doctor there for 41 years, it certainly seems as if the instinct to return to one's roots must have been very strong inside me. One acquaintance told me I had the reversionary migratory instinct normally reserved for the bird population. I soon discovered that many of my contemporaries did not share this enthusiasm for Stamford Hill and, even worse, felt that the presence of so many Chasidic Jews, from whom they thought they had made their escape, was embarrassingly uncomfortable. Frequently, remarks such as, "Isn't it awful having to be among all those people with their funny way of dressing?" or even worse, "They all seem to smell of gefilte fish" (a traditional dish of chopped fish, boiled with onion and served cold). My own experience was quite different. As I grew to know them better (or perhaps, more accurately, be re-introduced to them), I realised what less prejudiced minds should have known: that they were a group of individuals in which all varieties of behaviour were manifest, but all sharing one single faith and religious belief. Also, the smell of gefilte fish could only be discerned on the few days when it was being cooked!

Hackney was, and still is, notorious for its poverty and inner-city decay, but Stamford Hill, to the north of the borough, was rather like an oasis in the middle of a desert. Perhaps reflecting the middle-class growth of the late 1920s and early 30s, the houses were large and semi-detached; the streets wide and often tree-lined. After the war, the middle-class Jewish population had been replaced by working and artisan class and many of the largest houses, previously occupied by the wealthy, had been knocked down to make way for council flats. Sadly, in more recent years even the council flats have come to have a hierarchy, some having been allowed to deteriorate into near slums, while others have been maintained with a dignity of their own.

I started practice in Stamford Hill in 1957 having joined a single-handed, but rather unwell, doctor, who himself had joined a single-handed doctor when he arrived in England as one of the first refugees from Nazi Germany in 1934. The original doctor had in turn been in the practice since before the First World War. I was delighted one day when a patient, an elderly gentleman, gave me as a gift his medical card showing his entitlement to treatment. He had carefully crossed out the name of the first and second doctor and added my name. The card was stamped when he first received it, the date being 1911, the first year of Lloyd George's insurance act. The card was of special interest since the back was full of rules and regulations by which the recipient of medical care had to abide or risk being fined half a crown (12.5p) for bad behaviour, or worse still, be struck off the list if the bad behaviour was repeated. The emphasis on what was best for the doctor to what was good for the patient gradually changed over the years and reached its zenith with John Major's patients' charter, which laid down the law in relation to the duties of the doctor to the patient. Later still the GMC jumped on the bandwagon and in their guidelines on good medical practice placed "being polite at all times" near the top of the agenda. Somehow, being a good doctor in the traditional sense of being a good diagnostician and managing the patient appropriately had lost some of its importance to being merely polite.

My introduction to Stamford Hill coincided with the arrival of what I later came to regard affectionately as "the three musketeers". These were three Rabbis from the Lubavitch foundation, who had been settled into the area to pave the way for a growing community, which over the following years grew very large indeed. One had responsibility for maintaining religious principles, one for the finances and the third for influencing non-believers to become devout believers. The Lubavitch were a group of Chasidic Jews who had a missionary spirit: not to convert non-Jews into Judaism, but to convert anyone born Jewish into a religious or orthodox Jew. It is not surprising that arguments have flourished on the subject of "What is a Jew?" Anyone with a Jewish mother is considered Jewish, unlike most other religions that believe a child follows the faith of one's father. (This is an example of how highly logical the Jewish religion is. Before the advent of DNA it was not possible to know for certain who one's biological father was, but the mother, by necessity, has to be the proven parent.) Perhaps because of their missionary zeal, the followers of Lubavitch are very much easier to get on with than other Chasidic groups, who tend to keep very much to themselves. On the other side of the coin, my argument with Lubavitch is that they have had too much influence over some young people who, on embracing the faith, have discarded their family, who may not have been able to live under the restrictions deemed necessary to live the orthodox life.

Over the years the movement in Stamford Hill grew greatly and many buildings were taken over or new ones built to house the rising population. I am often asked if any of this community were my patients, and my answer is they made up about 30% of the numbers in the practice – but gave us 60% of the workload.

New recruits to the practice, both undergraduate students and post graduate registrars or partners, quickly came to realise that standards of practice had to remain high if one was to maintain the trust and confidence of the patient. So-called "British phlegm" and traditions of acceptance, even when wrong decisions were made, was not recognised by our patients. If you did not do the right thing, you were soon made aware of your failings, and were expected to keep going until the correct solution was found. I have on occasions been flattered to be informed that our practice had a high reputation and was one of the best in the area. I hope this is true, but if it is, no small part is due to having to keep up to the standards that our patients demanded.

Another habit, that could be annoying until one understood the reasoning behind it, was the demand for a second opinion. I soon came to learn that this was not meant as an insult to the doctor, but part of the orthodox Jewish culture was never to take a decision on what course to follow in life without first seeking the opinion and advice of a rabbi. Added to this was the difficulty caused by the diktat that once a rabbinical opinion had been given it became law, and one could not seek the opinion of another rabbi. In other words, the rabbi could trump the doctor's opinion, but the doctor could not, in turn, trump the rabbi. If the problem appeared to be a major one, it was likely that the most senior rabbi's opinion would be sought, who, in the case of most of our patients, was the Lubavitch rabbi, Rabbi Schneerson, a saintly figure who resided in New York and who was reputed to be an expert on every problem presented to him. He was greatly revered, and on his death it was found almost impossible to find someone wise enough to succeed him. It slowly dawned on me that when his advice was sought on medical matters, his usual response was: "Get a second opinion." The logic for this was not always easy to fathom, and it led to some rather bizarre situations, the most memorable being the occasion when I was interrupted from enjoying a half-day rest by a phone call asking me to attend the local A&E department to give a second opinion on a three-year-old patient of mine who had been admitted following a ghastly accident in which she had put her hand in a mincing machine, which was then turned on. The fingers and hand were in a bad condition, and could not be extricated without risk of losing the hand. The hospital advised an operation under full anaesthesia, explaining the risks involved. Not surprisingly the parents, in their agony, sought advice from the highest rabbinical authority, namely Rabbi Schneerson in New York. A hasty phone call received the reply "seek a second opinion" and as I was the child's medical practitioner, that duty fell to me. On arriving at the hospital I was met, not as I had expected by the casualty officer, but by a consultant general surgeon, consultant orthopaedic surgeon and anaesthetist all of who had already been involved and given advice. It did not take long for us all to agree that on this occasion the GP could advise the specialists and the operation should go ahead. The outcome was not as bad as it might have been, the child over the years recovering much of the use of her hand with the loss of one or two fingers.

Before leaving the subject of the wisdom and paternalism of the Lubavitch Rabbi, I must relate one other anecdote. After about 10 years in the practice, one of my patients, with whom I got on very well, came to see me. Usually we had a chat about our mutual religious community whenever she consulted me with one or other of her rapidly expanding family. On this particular occasion she could not wait to tell me: "Dr. Carne, you have arrived within the community." "Why, what have I done?" I asked. "I had need to ring the Rabbi in New York about medical advice you gave me, and his first question was, 'Who gave you this advice?' When I told him you had, he said: 'In that case you can go ahead and accept his advice.'" Touched as I was by the confidence installed in me, I think she was even more excited than I was. On a less happy note, I remember a young man hobbling in to see me about an injury to his foot. As his story unfolded, I found myself once again surprised at how in this day and age such reverence could be given to a fellow human being. His story was that he travelled to New York especially to visit the Rabbi (this was a common excursion, rather like the fervour that drives

Muslims to Mecca or Catholics to Lourdes) and having arrived at this crowded room where many other pilgrims were gathered, he noted that several were rushing to stand on a table to get a better view of the Rabbi as he entered the room. Unfortunately he did not notice that his foot was under one of the table legs and bore the brunt of the weight of 16 or so young men; he felt it would be disrespectful to move while the audience was taking place, so had to grin and bear the pain. By the time he arrived back in England and I saw him he had a very nasty injury indeed that took several months to finally heal.

On the rare occasions when I think about religion, and its importance to me personally, and the possible influence it has had on my life, I have concluded that while being intensely proud of my heritage, I do not feel in any accepted sense of the word "religious". To take it one stage further, I am not even certain whether I should consider myself an atheist or an agnostic. I think I am more inclined to the latter, but cannot help but be reminded of what that great raconteur and well-known surgeon, Dickson Wright, used to preach. He said that religion was no more than an insurance policy people took out for where they would end up after they died. He concluded by saying, with tongue firmly in cheek, (I paraphrase) "and I can't help wishing that I could be there when they arrive and find they have signed up to the wrong insurance company!"

For these reasons I could never completely enter into the life of my orthodox patients, but was happy to live among them as their medical adviser. I think to a certain degree they accepted me more readily in this role, recognising that I was empathetic to their needs, but not having to feel too guilty if they needed me to advise them on matters not altogether in keeping with their religious beliefs. If they felt they needed medical attention either on a Sabbath or festival, they did not feel too guilty about calling upon me, although on one occasion, the reverse was true. On the day before one of the festivals (*Yom Tovim*) I was called to see the wife of one of the more influential members of the orthodox community.

She had had a miscarriage with quite severe bleeding and I advised bed rest and told her I would come the next day to see how she was getting on. This made her husband very unhappy and he pointed out to me that as it was a *Yom Tov* I should not be working, and certainly should not use a car. I explained to him that I considered it was a medical necessity for her to be seen and I therefore intended to visit in spite of his protestations. He then played unfair, in my view. He invoked the name of my grandfather, about whom I have spoken previously. "Is it true," he said, "that your grandfather was Mendel Chaikin?" When I answered yes he responded: "What would he say if he knew he had such a *lobbas* (rascal) for a grandson?" Our mutual sense of humour, and recognition of the medical needs of his wife, came to our rescue, and we both laughed. I visited while he was away at synagogue, and his wife, fortunately, made a complete recovery.

If one was to survive in this religious environment, one had to learn to adapt to the whims and ways of the community. They were not ways that I was used to, but I learnt with necessary speed so did not make too many blunders. I knew the names of all the festivals and those when work was allowed and those when none was tolerated. I also was fairly cognisant with the hierarchy of the festivals, the Day of Atonement and *Shabbat* being at the top of the list. On *Chanukah*, the festival of lights, normal work could be carried out. On one occasion I was truly caught out when one of my lady patients came to see me and remarked on how quiet the surgery was. She was from abroad and had quite a strong accent, and when she remarked, "I suppose it is because it is the first day of *heretzal*", I was flummoxed. *Heretzel* I had not heard of, and wondered if I had heard her correctly. She repeated what she said, but slightly louder. (It is not only the English that believe if you speak loudly enough, you will be understood.) "What festival is *heretzel*?" I asked. She then remembered the second rule of being understood when speaking a foreign language, namely to speak both loudly and slowly. This time she was very precise as she slowly repeated: "Not *heretzel*–Harrods sale!" She had surmised correctly that many patients had deserted us to attend the famous sale.

English law is divided between statute (as laid down by parliament) and case law (as interpreted by judges). Similarly Jewish law, by which the orthodox community live, is determined by statute, or that which had been laid down by God and conveyed through Moses. They have to be obeyed and never questioned, whereas rabbinical law – which has been laid down through the ages and in theory open to interpretation and change, but in practice rarely, if ever, altered – is not immutable. I do know that there are 613 statutes, not because I have studied the subject but because a smart and very expensive kosher restaurant opened in the West End some years ago and was called 613. Most people, I understand, believed this to be the street number of the restaurant; in reality it represents the total number of statutes given by God to Moses.

I observed many anomalies in the efforts made by the local community to live up to the traditional orthodoxy of their forebears. While it is not too difficult to accept the clothes they copied from those favoured by the aristocracy of early 18th century Poland and Russia, and by which the community can still be recognised today, modern technology has produced as many questions as it has answers to the perennial question: "What exactly constitutes work, which must not be performed on certain days of the year?" A light may not be manually turned on, but a time switch is acceptable. Some accept that a refrigerator can be used on the Sabbath, but not if a light goes on, as it usually does, when the door is opened. (And what is the answer if the bulb is taken out?)

Another observation I have made over the years is whereas my parents' generation frequently rebelled against the orthodoxy of their parents, very few of the generation to which my patients belonged appeared to feel this need. Children and grandchildren of my patients appeared to be happy within the restrictions imposed by their elders, and the narrow way of life that the orthodoxy created. I well remember being somewhat surprised when a young child of about five years of age was being naughty in my presence and was threatened by his mother that if he didn't behave himself she would "not let him go to *shul* (synagogue) on Saturday". I was even more surprised when he immediately quietened down and did everything asked of him. Whether right or wrong, the conclusion I have reached is that the difference was in the school they attended. My parents, for better or worse, went to local English schools: their Jewishness was recognised but they observed the so-called British way of life, and found it a more attractive proposition. The orthodox community, as with other religions, have recognised this danger and defended against it by creating their own schools working to their own rules. Added to this, modern-day facilities such as television and newspapers are banned from the home, so that only the prescribed way of life is experienced, and dissatisfaction with it is minimal. A further consequence of this way of life has been that the children are brought up, and see themselves, as separate from the rest of the community. Not only do many speak with a foreign accent, but they are also like a foreign element within the country of their birth or adoption. This, of course, applies to other religions where the fundamentalist elements have wielded the most influence, in some cases with disastrous consequences.

A noticeable feature of the orthodox community is their propensity to very large families, and in our practice it was not unusual for there to be between 12 and 16 children in the same family. Many times I would see a lady for an antenatal examination, for her to be followed in by her pregnant daughter, also for an antenatal examination. I never reached the height of seeing a grandchild for an antenatal at the same clinic, but I believe it might have been just possible. The large family size was not accidental. After the years of the holocaust during the 1930s and 40s, in which six million Jews died at the hands of the Nazis, there was a strong instinct aimed at recovery of the lost generations. The religious laws of Judaism, by which the orthodox community strictly abided, not only forbade contraception, but unlike the Catholic religion, with their equally strict prohibitions, the Talmudic laws of cleanliness actively encouraged successful pregnancy as an outcome of intercourse. Under these laws, a woman is considered to be unclean while she is menstruating and for seven days after the completion of any vestige of bleeding. Elaborate means are employed to ensure that all bleeding has ceased, likely to be about seven days after the period has commenced. During this period of roughly two weeks, there must be no physical contact between husband and wife whatsoever, but at the end of the clean seven days she goes to the *mikvah*, or ritual bath, after which it is her duty to have sexual union with her husband. At this point you have a scenario in which the husband has had no physical contact with his wife: masturbation, or as it is fancifully referred to, onanism, is forbidden under the edict of wasted seed, and a testosterone-filled male is faced with a duty to make love to his wife, who herself has suffered similar privations over the previous two weeks. Stoking the flames of this highly charged sexual scenario is the medical fact that the average female would have arrived at the time of ovulation within her menstrual cycle. The circumstances are optimal for fertilisation and a new pregnancy. Occasionally there would be an obvious hiatus between, say, child number six and child number seven, the likely cause being that the woman had delayed going to the ritual bath for a week or so, thus missing the optimal time for fertilisation. On rare occasions my medical advice might be sought and I did not find it difficult to advise a woman who had had several births at short intervals that her body needed a rest, at least temporarily. She would then have to seek the rabbi's permission to allow her to have short-term contraceptive advice. Since the rabbi's word was final, it became fairly common knowledge which rabbis would be more sympathetic to the request. If contraceptive permission was granted, certain forms were more acceptable than others. Male condoms were, in my experience, never allowed, but female caps might be, the rationale being that with a male condom the sperm had no chance of reaching the womb, whereas with a cap it might. Usually the contraceptive pill was the method chosen, which had the added advantage that it could be said to be used as a means of regularising an irregular cycle.

As with all religions, miracles and magic are elements of religious faith. One example of this belief came to my attention when a very intelligent young woman informed me that I was wrong in my scientific belief in respect of her brother. The background was that her brother had had two daughters who developed normally, but then had two sons who appeared normal at birth, with no detectable defects, but at the ages of between one and two years had began to deteriorate with muscular dystrophy, and both had died by the age of three. They then had another daughter who grew to normal childhood. Although for various reasons, both medical and religious, there had been no autopsies performed and therefore no proof, I was quite certain that the tragedy could be explained medically on genetic grounds, the sex linking genes being well recognised. My patient was keen, she told me, to put the record straight and although she knew about my theory, it was wrong and the real reason was quite different. She then related to me the story, unknown to me, of how her brother had been engaged to be married to another woman, but had – very unusually in this community – broken off the engagement and married someone else. However he had not, as he should have done, sought the permission of a rabbi to break off his engagement and therefore had been "punished" by losing his two sons. After the second death, he had been advised to visit a rabbi in Israel for guidance, and had been advised to seek the forgiveness of the jilted woman, which he duly did. Having been granted forgiveness, he was then allowed to have another child that lived. This story was related to me while I had a student with me at the consultation, and she was greatly impressed, but I do not know whether the experience was soon forgotten or has stayed with her during her professional life. Certainly it gave me cause for thought.

Most conversions to Judaism among the population in which I live, rather than work, are for the purposes of marriage. It is not uncommon for the converting spouse, having undergone a vigorous indoctrination before being admitted to Judaism, to want to live a more orthodox life than the "born Jewish" member: this has led to problems. Within the Stamford Hill community, the few conversions I came across were of people with a strong faith in God who had concluded that Judaism was the only way of accepting this truth. One such lady, a highly intelligent woman with a PhD, answered my question to her "What do you find the most difficult thing to accept, living the ultra-orthodox life?" by stating, after some thought, "Well, to tell the truth, the only thing I find really hard is not thinking about God when I am on the toilet." An honest, but wholly unexpected response, but further proof that the really difficult-to-achieve things in life are those forbidden to us.

To conclude this chapter about a community that were so much a part of my life for so many years, I would say that it was an experience for which I am thankful. They have taught me a degree of tolerance towards others who do not believe as I do, but have more faith in their beliefs, and with whom a strong relationship can survive. If only the world could learn the same lesson.

CHAPTER XVIII

TV Radio and Stages

As well as that part of my make up that attracted me to medicine, I have always recognised that lurking inside, somewhere, was a desire to display my thespian nature. The two came together whenever I had the occasional opportunity to appear on television and be heard on radio. Each time it gave me the desire for more of the same; but over the years I had a limited number of appearances, with which my ego had to be satisfied.

I was still at school and aged about 16 when a radio producer decided he wanted to produce Eliot's *Murder in the Cathedral* and have a cast of schoolchildren to act as the chorus. I was one of the chosen few and felt very important chanting my one line together with about 20 other schoolboys. A humble beginning, perhaps, but when a couple of years later, in 1946, I went on a school trip to Hilversum in Holland I felt very experienced in the art of broadcasting and was once again successful in being chosen to be spokesman for our party when the local radio station decided to broadcast a programme about us. It was only one year since the war had ended and Holland, like so much of Europe, had suffered terribly at the hands of the German invasion forces. Coming from Britain we were looked at with envy, but from our point of view it was difficult to appreciate the extent of the deprivation they had experienced. Transport was running, the people looked well fed again, and we ate at least as well as we did in the still-rationed England from where we had travelled. The broadcast consisted of me and one or two others being interviewed about our own experiences during the war: compared with theirs, ours sounded very banal. Hearing myself talk on the radio, and a foreign service to boot, once again made me feel very important.

My next fling with the media was about 30 years later: in 1977 or thereabouts. Something contentious was happening in the NHS – I cannot remember what it was, but the NHS has not been short of contentious issues in the 60 years it has been in existence. The health correspondent of the *Evening Standard* had been given my name as someone who might have views on the issue (as, of course, I did – views on issues are something in which I am a specialist and never short of!). I remember him asking me at the end of the interview how long I had been practising in London and I told him it was exactly 20 years. "So you are not a novice, then," was his response. In the quoted article I was actually described as the "experienced GP from Hackney". I was not to know that 20 years was less than half the time I was destined to practice in Hackney.

Practicing in Hackney was the source of another experience that I remember with some amusement. My brother (also a GP and involved with the media even more than I was) appeared in a TV programme about health. On the occasion in question the programme involved a dermatologist and a GP whose role was to ask the questions and, if given the opportunity, put the GP's point of view on the subject. The subject that night was acne, not very easily controlled by the treatments then available. My brother asked the requisite questions to which he received suitable replies. A few day's later I was surprised to be told by my receptionist that an appointment had been made for me to see a young lady from the north of England. They had insisted that they wanted to see me and that no error had been made. Feeling both flattered and curious I was surprised to see that my patient was a young girl of about 14 and her mother, both with very broad Lancashire (or perhaps Yorkshire) accents. I noticed that the young girl was very spotty, but thought no more of it. I asked what the problem was and how they had come to know my name. My flattered feeling collapsed, when they replied, "We saw the programme on television the other evening and as our own doctor has not helped my daughter's spots, we came to London, rang the BMA and asked who 'the acne doctor' was, and they gave your name."

Another example, perhaps, how northern and cockney accents are separated only by a common language, as Shaw might have said.

Between about 1980 and 1995, I became one of the names on the list of GPs to approach for views on one or other aspect of a rapidly changing health service. One enormous reform came about in 1991, when the Conservative party, under the health secretaryship of Kenneth Clarke, introduced fundholding into primary care. I will be writing separately about this elsewhere, but for this chapter, it is necessary to say that due to my involvement as a "first-wave" fundholder, and my enthusiasm for it, I was interviewed on several occasions on the emerging system, about which there was much publicity, most of it bad. I tried hard to redress the balance – but anyway it is now history, the newly elected Labour party kicking the scheme into touch in 1998 for no good reason that I can see, other than that the Tories had introduced it. Many of these interviews were conducted in my surgery, one or two at conferences I attended, or in a TV studio. I very quickly learned two important techniques when being interviewed. If they were to be recorded it was more relaxing and less nerve racking, but the interview suffered very badly from editing. What was finally shown on screen tended to be more the producer's view of what you were trying to say rather than what was important to oneself. I came to prefer the live interviews: although the tension and anxiety levels were much higher, and one had to be careful of what was said and how it was said, at least there could be no changes to what you were trying to put across. The other technique I learned from watching the politicians: whatever the question and however complicated it appeared to be, start by saying, "That is a very important question, but before answering it, I would just like to say . . ." and then state what you want to get across. This technique only really works when it is a live broadcast, otherwise your contribution is unlikely to see the light of day.

On the whole I found the distraction from my normal work both stimulating and interesting, and I came to learn about the power of television. Even the most mundane programmes are viewed by numbers that any theatre would give their eyeteeth to emulate. One interesting programme in which I participated on two occasions was *The Midnight Hour*. It went out live at midnight and consisted of a panel of four plus a chairman. Over a period of half an hour or so various topics of the day were discussed. I found it particularly interesting since the other participants were mostly politicians, ranging from unknowns to ministers of state. It is with nostalgia, tinged with pride, that I can now say I appeared on television with many of the bright lights of today's political scene (and some for whom the lights have dimmed again). Amongst others were Charles Kennedy, Tessa Jowel, and Ian Duncan-Smith. In view of the late hour it was broadcast I had doubts that anyone watched it at all, so on the second occasion I appeared, while in the so-called green room enjoying the BBC hospitality of a glass of plonk and crisps, I asked the producer how many viewers the show had. He admitted that in TV terms the number was small, no more than 250,000. Later, on thinking this over, I calculated that this was probably about the same number that had seen the play *The Mousetrap*, which had been showing in one of London's smallest West End theatres for over 50 years. Looked at in this way, one's mind can only boggle at the thought of the power a show with an audience of several million must have. In passing I might add that in comparison with the enormous amount of money I've learned the BBC pay some of the better known names, the £60 (plus transport to and from the studio) seems a little mean in hindsight.

One other programme in which I was involved on two occasions was called *Hypotheticals*. I found this a fascinating concept, in which about 12 or 14 experts in various fields sat round a table and a moderator then proceeded to outline a scenario before asking members of the panel how they would have reacted to the situation. The catch was that having answered the question "entirely to your own satisfaction" the moderator would then add another dimension to the story in an attempt to throw you off balance. In spite of this, it did replicate real life more than a dramatised production might have done. This was an opportunity to make an utter fool of oneself unless you kept wide awake and tried not to be led into an impossible hypothetical situation. Great fun to do and very interesting to watch, and with the added advantage of being live.

I still maintained an interest in the theatre, mainly as something to watch, but I also enjoyed my association over a period of about 20 years with amateur dramatics. A friend was actively involved in an amateur theatrical group called the Charities Theatre Group. They wrote and produced both revues and musicals, many of the latter being parodies of more famous West End musicals. Examples of the shows produced were *My Fair Sadie, Morrie of Arabia* and *The Teitlebaum File*. They mainly appealed to Jewish audiences, especially those that either came from or harboured an empathy with the East End and North London environs where they had been brought up. The shows were of a very high amateur standard and were performed on Sunday nights over a period of two to three months at various major London theatres. All proceeds went to charity and quite enormous sums were raised. The leading actor in the shows was the late Alf Fogel. He was a very funny man who not only acted in but also part-wrote the shows. An obituary in *The Times* described him as "the British equivalent of Billy Crystal or Mel Brooks" – high praise indeed. I became the honorary medical officer for the group and enjoyed my association both during rehearsals and actual performances. It was interesting to watch the participants over the years, who showed a great reluctance to give up the roles to which they were suited as young men and women but had, over the years, became less and less suited as their true age overcame their stage ages by several factors. However, to me the shows stayed funny and I had many laughs over the years.

I have always had a secret desire to be asked to appear on the famous radio show *Desert Island Discs*. I am well aware that the chances of my receiving such an invitation are nil, but it has occurred to me that I can satisfy my fantasy by writing about my requests, and the reasons for them. This has the added advantage of letting me be as self-indulgent as I wish. Having harboured the wish for some time, I have also had time to plan how I would approach the task in my mind. Now I can put it on paper.

I have no doubt I would divide my choices of music into periods of my life and the associations that accompany them. Shakespeare only managed to describe seven ages of man, but I have the luxury of eight: I am not sure whether that makes it easier or harder.

For choice number one, I return to my childhood: these were the years that led up to the declaration of World War Two in September 1939, at which time I was nearly 11 years old. My father was a keen football supporter and had been a regular spectator at Clapton Orient (now Leyton Orient) since he had been a schoolboy. Quite often he would take my brother and me along with him and on these occasions we would arrive home just before 5pm, a time at which there was a regular band show on the radio by Bert Ambrose and his orchestra. My father always said he had been at school with him, so he felt almost like family, even though I never actually met him. As well as being one of the leading orchestra leaders of the day (Henry Hall, Billy Cotton, and Harry Roy were others) he also had a great gift of spotting talent. Two of his lady singers were Anne Shelton and Vera Lynne, the former being probably the better singer, but with less of what would now be known as "X-factor". Vera Lynne, who is still a household name and indeed a Dame, was the forces' sweetheart during the war. Who does not remember "There'll be bluebirds over the white cliffs of Dover" and "We'll meet again" even to this day? Amazingly, in 2009, she achieved the distinction, in her late eighties, of being number one in the pop music charts for the songs she had sung during the war. Truly, "what goes round comes round".

For my first piece of music, and to remind me of those early years of my life, I would choose a number played fairly frequently at the time, "The Teddy Bears' Picnic". I am sure that childhood memories, which are nearly all good, the bad having been largely sublimated by the passage of time, would come flooding back at the first bars. If there is still a record of it available by Ambrose and his orchestra, so much the better.

Choice number two would encompass my secondary school days, which coincided with the war years. From the beginning of the war until 1942 I was evacuated to Northampton, about which I have written in another chapter. My parents then felt it was safe enough (and presumably were missing me enough) to bring me back to London. As a means to improve the morale of the nation regular lunchtime concerts were given at the National Gallery in Trafalgar Square. I do not remember by whom I was first introduced to them, but I do remember attending about half a dozen in all and being blown over by the atmosphere, music and, if the weather was fine, sitting after the concert on the steps of the gallery overlooking Trafalgar Square, eating a sandwich lunch. Among others, famous artists such as the pianists Myra Hess and Solomon, and the conductor and composer Michael Tippet, all gave personal performances. This was really my first introduction to the beauty of classical music and there are so many pieces that would invoke one of the happier memories I have of what was really a very fraught time. Because the setting of the recitals lent itself to the intimacy of chamber music, it is from this genre that I would make my choice. Any quartet by Haydn would be suitable.

Choice number three would help me remember my days at school. I was fortunate to attend a very progressive (for the time) co-educational grammar school. Pupils came from a very mixed cultural background but were not as ethnically assorted as they were later to become. While morning prayers were proceeding in the main assembly hall those of us who did not attend, usually on religious grounds, were left to ourselves in a classroom, the responsibility for what we did being our own. At least once a week we ran a music circle and would take it in turn to bring along a "78" vinyl record to play on a wind up gramophone, and talk about what we had played. It was quite eclectic and the music ranged from jazz to classics. Wanting to be different when my turn for presentation came, I found a jazz record involving mainly a plucked double bass, called "The Big Noise from Winnetka". (Does anyone remember it now?) Because I also considered myself rather too highbrow to play such a lowly piece, I decided to hide my philistine side by introducing the record in a literal French translation as "*Le Grand Bruit de Winnetka*". It was halfway through the first side before anyone twigged that it was not a piece of high classical music in the baroque style. This record should be sufficient to bring back memories of some of what should have been "the best days of my life".

At the age of about 14 I decided to explore classical music more extensively. As I have no actual musical ability, I made a conscious decision to listen to as much classical music that I could make time for. As part of this discipline, I attended a recital at the Wigmore Hall. It was a piano recital, but I no longer remember the name of the artist. Studying the programme I noted that the second piece was a piano sonata by Beethoven under the title "The Waldstein Sonata". For some reason the first piece played was very short and I have no memory of it at all, but suddenly the pianist was playing the opening bars of the sonata and my whole being became aware of the music in a way that I have not experienced since. It is not played as often as the better-known sonatas of Beethoven such as "The Appassionato" or "The Moonlight" but it remains my favourite and would certainly be my choice for record number four.

I have now presented half of my choices and it is time to grow up. Choice number five reminds me of what was to turn out to be the most significant event of my life, namely first meeting my future wife, Pearl. I was 16, and the relationship has lasted over 68 years. If I were to be allowed only one choice this would be it, not because it is my favourite piece of music, but because it represents the commencement of the rest of my life. August 6th 1945 was a very auspicious day; the war in Europe had come to a victorious end, but Japan remained a menace to civilisation as we knew it. The allies decided to speed up the capitulation of Japan by dropping a new form of weapon, the so-called atom bomb. Its effects were catastrophic and the world has lived in a state of high anxiety that it might be used again ever since. Whatever history has to record as to the rights or wrongs of using such a powerful tool, at the time there was a great sense of relief that an ending to the war was a definite possibility. The cruelty of the Japanese at that time and their culture of "no surrender at any price" was legendary; the conditions under which the troops were fighting, and perhaps even worse, the prisoners of war were suffering, meant that the majority of people felt the correct decision had been made and the enormous loss of life suffered by the Japanese in Hiroshima was worth while. As history will recall it took a second atom bomb on Nagasaki a few days later (perhaps with less justification) for the Japanese to finally surrender. What history will not recall is my own personal "Hiroshima" experience – meeting Pearl –, which occurred a day later, on the 7th August 1945. The uncle of a school friend had become engaged to a young lady who had three younger sisters. They had lived in the country during the war, and as teenagers had experienced very little of London life. One of them had been invited to spend a fortnight with the family of my friend and I suggested that I should ask a girl to make up a foursome to attend the National Ballet, which at that time had their home in Sadler's Wells theatre. We were both keen balletomanes and we would go early in the morning and for sixpence obtain a stool that reserved our place in the queue for the gallery (which cost a further shilling). These were the great days of Margot Fonteyn, Beryl Grey, Moira Shearer and Robert Helpman, and I was in love with all of them (except Helpman!). Having agreed the arrangements and found a young lady to accompany me, I set up the stools and returned in the early evening to meet up with my friend and his country visitor. I remember two things from that evening: the ballet "Les Sylphides" (made up from the music of Chopin) and the emotional upheaval I felt on seeing Pearl for the first time. This is not meant to be a love story, so I will not go into this any further, but the Chopin Nocturne which opens the ballet will be sufficient to let me contemplate the blessings that have arisen as a result of our meeting.

Choice number six beckons. Another significant period in my life was the time I spent as a medical student at the London Hospital. I was keen on amateur dramatics and had played in two productions while at school: I was the Roman Legionnaire in *Androcles and the Lion* and Sergius in *Arms and the Man*, both by George Bernard Shaw. At the time I played Sergius, who is an overblown, blustering, "chocolate box" soldier, there was a London production of the same play with the great Laurence Olivier playing the name part. I went to see it, and afterwards tried my best, not very successfully, to copy his interpretation. Unsuccessful or not, it was great fun doing it. The competition for parts at the London Hospital was more difficult and to my disappointment the production that was to be performed was the Gilbert and Sullivan opera *HMS Pinafore*. As I have already said, I have no musical ability, and this includes (in trumps) my singing voice. Singing in tune has always been impossible (I have noted that when I do sing, in my head it sounds like Frank Sinatra, but what comes out my mouth is a foghorn). But I did want to be in the production, so in the end I "sang" in the chorus – well, not exactly sang, but mouthed the words while others did the singing. I don't think anyone noticed. So record number six chooses itself; something from *HMS Pinafore*, and in view of my feigned involvement, why not the opening chorus. "We are mighty men and true . . ."

Number seven has to reflect my air force days. I have written about this so will not say anything more here, but for a piece of music it must be William Walton's march from *The Dam Busters*.

Finally I come to choice number eight. This is more difficult, since having overindulged myself in the earlier years it has to represent the rest of my life up to the present. My taste in the arts is fairly eclectic and I enjoy drama, the opera and good musicals. For my final piece I will acknowledge musical theatre rather than opera. My first experience of the great musicals was *Oklahoma*, to which I was introduced by Pearl who had discovered its joys even before I discovered her. Recently I have been very disappointed in the tendency that musicals have of either being full of songs requiring the cast to raise their arms in homage and belt out the final line in order to encourage the audience to stand up and cheer, or being stories written around the words of songs from various pop groups. However, one composer has more than filled the gap left by the past masters including Cole Porter, Irving Berlin, Rogers and Hammerstein, Lerner and Lowe and, of course, Leonard Bernstein. I refer to Stephen Sondheim, of whom I am a great fan. It is from one of his musicals that I will choose my final record, especially as it represents the art world as well as the musical. *Sunday in the Park with George* is a brilliant musical, built round that famous painting by the pointist Georges Seurat, "A Sunday Afternoon on the Island of La Grande Jatte". I think the most suitable title is the theme song of the show, "Putting it Together", which is what I have tried to do in this chapter.

Guests on *Desert Island Discs* are allowed one luxury and one book to accompany them as castaways. My luxury would have to be a large television set with as many DVDs to show on it as I would be allowed (choosing eight of these would make another chapter!). As for a book, I think a volume containing the complete works of Anthony Trollope would keep me well occupied.

So I have arrived at the end of my dream. It has amused me to compose it, but I have no doubt that on another day my choice might have been different (with the exception of number five!) My task completed, I will now float away from the sleepy lagoon of fantasy, and back to reality.

CHAPTER XVIV

A Funny Thing Happened
on the Way . . .

Let us call her Beryl: she was a small bird-like "professional" spinster with a very precise, but quiet, voice to which one was forever saying, "Pardon?" Shyness oozed out of her, so any attempt at more than the most superficial examination was a herculean task, which, I am ashamed to say, was sometimes only observed in the breach. On this occasion it very quickly became obvious that halfway measures would not be enough. She was complaining of a cough, productive of a "nasty coloured phlegm" (her words). Checking her temperature, pulse and throat did not present a problem, but I was well aware that on this occasion examination of her chest was a must. As it was mid-winter and very cold, I was not surprised, but somewhat disheartened, that this would involve removing several layers of clothes: a daunting prospect for both of us. I asked her to go behind the curtains and remove her top things so I could examine her. After a suitable interval of about two minutes – it seemed more like half an hour – I picked up my stethoscope and invaded her privacy behind the curtains. As I had half feared, she had acceded to my request only insofar as she had removed her overcoat, scarf and cardigan. Her blouse remained fully buttoned up to the neck. I asked her to take off her blouse and in an effort to speed up the process I stayed with her, hoping this might encourage her to stick to the task in hand. Turning away from me, she began unbuttoning her blouse, starting at the top and working her way all the way down to the last button. The blouse then had to be pulled out of the skirt and slowly removed. I was confronted by a long-sleeved vest, which turned out to be only an over-vest, and after its laborious removal, an under-vest was exposed. I suppose that the actual time it took to get to this stage was probably no more than a few minutes, but with the awareness of a busy morning ahead and several people still waiting to be seen, plus several visits to be carried out after surgery was finished, it seemed that several hours had passed. I am not normally an insensitive man, but I must confess that by this time valour overtook discretion and I felt that a little help would speed up the process. (I was well aware that after completing the examination the whole process would have to be reversed as she dressed up again.) In an effort to remove her under-vest, which I assumed was the last layer of clothing, I took hold of it in order to pull it over her neck and yanked it upwards, only to be greeted by a loud and very high-pitched scream emanating from her. The cause of her discomfort quickly became apparent as I realised she was actually wearing what used to be called (when I was a child) coms, or combinations. For those too young to remember the garment, it was an all-in-one vest and knickers, buttoned at the front and back to allow for necessary body functions, but not designed to be removed by pulling over one's head. Try to imagine the picture, and you will understand why it took me a very long time for embarrassment at the memory to turn to amusement: even as I write this, some 40 years after the event, I can still feel my cheeks turning a deep red.

Over the years, the number of patients who liked to remind me "I was your first patient" grew in number. If everyone with this dubious claim to fame had, in fact, been the first patient I saw, the queue would have stretched from the surgery at Stamford Hill to Stoke Newington. Fanny Mandelstein (not her name but henceforward to be called just Fanny) really was, if not the first, certainly one of the very early patients whom I was privileged to look after for many years. She was a delightful and very kind woman and already, when I first knew her, an archetypical *booba* (Jewish grandmother). Unfortunately she had only one son and as he had no children she was not an actual grandma, which was probably one reason why she took such a kindly interest in my own two daughters, who were very young when she first became aware of their presence. No consultation with her would be allowed to terminate without an enquiry as to their well-being, and I was very willing to talk about them. I must have told her on one occasion the dates of their birthdays, because from then on when their birthday came round there was always a birthday card from her, more often than not with a £5 note inside to "buy them something nice". She had a great sense of humour, of an old fashioned East End nature. I hope I helped her feel better whenever she saw me, because she certainly put me in a good mood after I had seen her.

I was surprised one day when she came into my surgery carrying a large shopping bag, obviously full but with no apparent groceries to be seen. It looked as if it was full of bits of old newspaper. I was still speculating on the contents when she sat down carefully and placed the carrier bag even more carefully down by her side. She was much less loquacious than usual and we seemed to get down to the nitty-gritty of her visit more quickly than was customary. Recognising the potential seriousness of the forthcoming consultation I immediately asked what had brought her to see me. Instead of a flood of explanation she merely put her hand up, meaning "Wait". Her next action was puzzling: she put her hand inside the carrier bag and removed one of the lumps of newspaper, which I could now see had something wrapped inside it. She replaced the bag on the floor and carefully and slowly undid the newspaper covering, revealing a flower-patterned bone china saucer, which she put down on the desk in front of me. Then she removed another, slightly larger, package of newspaper. The pattern of uncovering the contents was repeated, but this time a matching cup was disclosed and placed on the desk next to the saucer. I watched transfixed as a third and final parcel was removed, and this time a teaspoon was uncovered and placed next to the cup. I was becoming somewhat frustrated as I saw my role in surgery as a healer rather than a dealer . . . "Yes, but why have you come to see me?" I exploded. Once again the hand went up and only one word was uttered: "Wait." As I sank lower in my seat, Fanny took the cup and placed it on the saucer and then took the teaspoon and placed it on the saucer next to the cup. Was this a hint that it was time I offered her a cup of tea or coffee? Had she taken leave of her senses? I could no longer contain myself. "This is all very well, but I do need to know what has brought you to see me," I said. I was a little ashamed as I recognised my voice had risen and my frustration might be interpreted by her as anger. At last I received an answer. Only one word from her, as slowly she leaned forward across the desk and picked up the combination cup, saucer and spoon. "Look," she said – and might have added "and listen", because the explanation for her odd behaviour became immediately clear. As she raised the cup etc from the table it shook and cluttered, demonstrating better than any words could the very obvious shaking of her right hand that she was unable to control. I don't think I have ever seen a better presentation of early Parkinsonism. A few weeks later when she came to see me about another matter, I reminded her of her rather bizarre but effective way of demonstrating her problem and how, on reflection, I had found it very amusing. "Oh, yes," she said, "I thought about it as well. I realise I should have brought some sugar and milk and we could have had a nice cup of tea together." Long since departed – but I loved Fanny dearly.

Jessie was quite another cup of tea (if you will pardon the metaphor). She was not a "heartsink" patient – she was a "heartsink in spades", proof of which could be found in her history of having been struck off the list of more GPs than any other patient in the whole of the borough. In those days GPs had the luxury of giving patients two weeks notice that they no longer could keep them on their list. This may have been for several reasons, such as the patient having moved out of the area or circumstances within the practice having changed, but it was also a method by which the doctor could call "feinites" when he felt he could no longer cope. As Jessie's address always remained the same, I assume it was the latter reason that was the cause of her numerous dismissals. In order to protect the rights of a patient, however difficult, to retain the services provided by the NHS, the controlling authority could allocate the patient to a practice, who would then have to accept them for a minimum period. This was the mechanism by which I found myself her medical adviser (well: GP, perhaps, since Jessie never accepted advice). One of the main problems, from the GPs point of view, was that Jessie would frequently request home visits for non-existent complaints, and to add insult to injury would more often than not be out taking the dog for a walk when one arrived. It was difficult to accept that she could walk further with her dog than the distance to the surgery. Coupled with her cavalier attitude to doctors, it was not surprising that the response from her various GPs in the past was unsympathetic.

In spite of all I had heard about her, I was determined to try and make our relationship better than it had been with her previous doctors. It was almost a test. Could I keep her as a patient longer than all the others had done? (Was hubris settling in?) The turning point in our relationship came when I was called to visit her yet again for no very obvious reason. When I arrived, she was just returning from a shopping trip, so I was, perhaps, a little angry and near, in fact, to abdicating my responsibility and joining the other GPs who had removed her from their lists. In my frustration I shouted at her: "You are a very naughty girl, but if you are good I can make you better." The look on her face, somewhere between disbelief and indignation at my outburst, very soon changed to one of recognition that she had perceived someone with feelings of anger that could match her own. "Why do you say that?" she asked in a voice much more submissive than I had heard from her previously. I then took ten valuable minutes to explain how her behaviour towards doctors was unacceptable and was the reason for her own inability to keep a doctor. Somewhere within this outburst, I must have inserted a joke because I recognised for the first time that we did have one thing, at least, in common: we both had a sense of humour and enjoyed a good joke. I then found myself making her an offer, which surprised me. I knew that she had a son who was a taxi driver, and I agreed to give her an hour-long consultation at my surgery, once a month. I would come in an hour early allowing her time to bring up any complaint she wished, as long as her son would bring her to see me. I offered that I would visit her at home if a neighbour or her son requested it, should they be worried. I actually went further inasmuch as I actually wrote to the health authority stating the above and asking for permission to see her as a non-NHS patient, but for whom I would make no charge; I asked to be allowed to issue her NHS prescriptions on the understanding that she would not actually be on my list (with all the restrictions and penalties to which I might be exposed). I was informed by return of post that there was no way that this would be allowed; but at least I had offered and would feel less guilty if the time came that I could stand it no longer.

Unexpectedly my offer worked very well. Her son, who I soon discovered found her as big a pain as all the rest of us, played along and brought her in his taxi at the pre-arranged time once a month. We discussed any medical problems she might have, but these turned out to be very minor and few in number. Much of the time was taken up trying to make each other laugh, but this became more onerous as the jokes ran out. However, it did drastically reduce the call outs to her and after about six months of the arrangement, my confidence was boosted when she walked in for her arranged consultation with a box of chocolates in her hands. I felt elated at the realisation (or so I thought) that my sacrifice was paying off and she was actually trying to say thank you. Deflation of my ego quickly followed when she placed the chocolates on my desk in front of me, with the request, "Please don't let me forget them when I go, I am taking them to a friend who has invited me for tea." My self-value suffered another dip when she brought me what appeared to be a half bottle of whisky saying, as she handed it over, "I have brought you a present today." This was followed by, "I passed it this morning – I am worried I might have sugar, so please test it for me."

The success I achieved with Jessie had a consequence when, after several years, she finally moved to live with her son. This was several miles away so I had no mixed feelings when I genuinely had to turn down her request to keep her on my books as I was the only doctor she had really ever got on with. I had succeeded in earning her trust, but on the down side, I had made her dependent on me. For about two years more I would receive a letter from her every six months or so: they would cover about five pages of small, closely knit writing, with every corner of the paper covered. After-thoughts would adorn any margins she found left over, leaving the whole letter almost meaningless. To those who are dragging at the bit to tell me there was probably a psychological reason for her behaviour, my answer is: "I know."

CHAPTER XX

When Things Go Wrong

To paraphrase Jane Austin, it is a truth universally acknowledged that the medical profession is caring, careful and compassionate. But like all truths, whether universally acknowledged or otherwise, there are bound to be exceptions. I am not talking about exceptions of Harold Shipman proportions, but about those where the relationship between doctor, as carer, and patient, as receiver of care, go awry. The commonest cause is lack of communication, but it also has to be said that another, and perhaps more fundamental, cause is either or both doctor and patient failing to recognise, or confusing, their roles in the interaction that occurs when a consultation takes place. The expectations by the patient of what the doctor can achieve may be too high, or the hopes of the doctor of what can be achieved be unreachable, but a more realistic understanding of the transaction would in many cases avoid the inevitable complaints that follow. I am reminded of a local colleague whose reputation among the local community was so high that many of them believed he was God: unfortunately he believed them.

My own experience of complaints involved those in which I was the complainant, those in which I was complained against, and those where colleagues were complained against and I had some involvement. I know the anger and frustration suffered by patients when things appear to have gone wrong and how these feelings become intensified when one is convinced of the justice of one's own case. Although it happened many years ago the memories of one such incident are still vivid to me. I was called out to visit a patient at about 9pm. She gave a history of being about 16 weeks pregnant and had suddenly started having severe abdominal pain and slight bleeding. She was in a lot of distress and I was fairly certain the diagnosis was "threatened miscarriage". (Miscarriages might be "threatening", "inevitable" or "missed".) I was equally certain she required admission to hospital in view of the length of the pregnancy and consequent potential for serious complications. I therefore arranged for her to be admitted to the local general hospital and requested an ambulance to take her there. To my intense surprise I was called by her husband the following morning at about 7am requesting an urgent visit as his wife was "in a dreadful state". I arrived to find a very distressed lady with a 16-week foetus lying at her side. I was told that after a cursory examination the hospital had told her to go home as the "miscarriage was not inevitable". She had no choice but to comply and shortly after arriving home she had entered into mini-labour which after several hours culminated in giving birth to the foetus. No pain relief or TLC had been offered by the hospital, and no attempt had been made to let me know that she had not been admitted. I considered this a disgraceful standard of care and in my anger wrote to the consultant under whose care I had admitted her, complaining about the behaviour of his junior staff. Instead of support, I received the reply that he had discussed the matter with his registrar who had seen the lady on admission and had found no evidence of a threatened miscarriage. He completely ignored the fact that within an hour or two she had an inevitable miscarriage followed by the actual miscarriage. He assured me he was a very good registrar who would not have made a mistaken diagnosis and that was the end of the matter. I felt I had no alternative but to make an official complaint on behalf of my patient.

When a complaint was made against me, years earlier, the feelings of anger and frustration were very similar. I was young and perhaps had a greater need to correct things I conceived as wrong. The case involved a middle-aged gentleman who worked for a government department as a clerk. He had impetigo, a skin infection causing multiple sores and boil-like lesions over the body. Fortunately, since the advent of antibiotics, it is usually quickly healed and not commonly seen nowadays.

I treated his condition with the appropriate antibiotic and cream and gave him a certificate to stay away from work. One week later the lesions had all dried up, were no longer infectious to others, and he would be, in my opinion, fit to return to work within a few more days. I gave him a final certificate to this affect. The next morning he returned to inform me that because of the scars from the scabs on his face, he was growing a beard to hide them: his manager had informed him that "a beard does not look nice while it is growing, so get a certificate to stay away from work until it is fully grown". I did not see this as a medical reason to pay someone public money, and therefore refused his request. The anger this response elicited surprised me, and I was both shocked and distressed to be informed a few weeks later that a complaint had been made and I would have to appear before a medical services committee to explain my actions. If found guilty (in other words, in breach of my terms of service) I could be warned about my behaviour, have a withholding from my pay or even, in extreme cases, be barred from working in the NHS. For a young doctor with a family to support this was a very distressing situation, and the reassurance from colleagues that it was most unlikely I would be found in breach only provided minimum reassurance. Although eventually I was not found in breach it took about nine months before the matter was cleared up. That was nine months of sleepless nights, waking up and trying to sort out in my mind how I would best justify my actions to a set of strangers. The reassurance from a senior member of the committee before whom I appeared that the reason it had gone so far was to show that "justice had to be seen to be done" did not make me feel any better, but it did leave me with a deep sense of sympathy when colleagues had to appear before the committee later on, especially if for fairly trivial reasons.

When I look back at these episodes, I realise that after many decades similar problems are still reported in the NHS, and that really nothing very much has changed.

On a lighter note, I remember another reprimand in which our practice was involved. Although one tends to think that difficulty in funding of the health service, and in particular the provision of drugs, is a recent phenomenon, in fact finding the finances to pay for all the medications demanded by patients has *always* been a problem. In the 1960s and early 70s one method used in an attempt to keep some control on the financial implications of prescribing was to average the cost of drugs for each individual practice, area by area. If a practice or practitioner went more than a certain percentage over the average figure (it was 30% or 50%, I cannot remember exactly) they could be called to account for their profligacy. One year we found ourselves some way above the average for our district, although it has to be said that inner city areas notoriously had very low averages: this might be judged as the standards of practice being either better or worse than the rest of the country, depending on how you looked at it. We received notification that we were to be visited by the local government medical officer, to "discuss our prescribing habits". Again, several weeks of anxiety, coupled with hours spent investigating possible reasons and justification for our figures. In the event, he turned out to be a very amiable doctor, who had spent several years in general practice. He had "heard it all before" and was not very impressed with my argument that research into our figures had shown that although our total cost was high, the average cost of each individual item we had prescribed was lower than the average. Also our average cost was no higher than the rest of the country. I tried to persuade him that the figures suggested that we were, in fact, prescribing more items because we were seeing more patients, and that was a sign of good doctoring rather than bad. He immediately pointed out that I had prescribed a more expensive, but user-friendly, ointment for patients complaining of haemorrhoids rather than the more mundane but equally effective cheaper preparation. "Why," he asked, "did you do that?" I suppressed the immediate response that came to mind – "My patients with piles are a pain in the butt" – and contented myself with the rather weak excuse that it was more pleasant to use. After about three hours of this cross between an inquisition and a music hall act, he sat back in his chair, lit his pipe (you could in those days) and made a wise and completely accurate statement. "I know you find this a waste of time, but I also know that you will not want to go through this whole process again in a hurry, so you will reduce your prescribing costs." He was so right!

I once attended a lecture on complaints against doctors given by a distinguished appeal court Judge. He made a point of repeating a dictum that I had heard many times before, that most patients when they make a complaint are only seeking an explanation and an apology. My experience of complaints was that with many complainants, once made, they wanted their pound of flesh: nothing less than punishment for the doctor and financial compensation for themselves would do. An apology by the doctor is not infrequently used as evidence of guilt, and although it is regrettable, it is one reason why lawyers or Defence Societies acting on behalf of a doctor will often advise them that silence is better. I had the temerity to stand up after his lecture and put over this point of view. I think it might have been the first time for many years that any judgment he gave had been questioned (other than by the House of Lords perhaps), and his caustic reply and withering looks lived with me for a long time.

Because doctors are also human, there are bound to be times when tempers flare or words are said that are regretted as soon as they have been pronounced. Personality clashes are inevitable and a personal dislike for some patients is also the norm. Recognising these negative feelings within oneself, I very early on came to the conclusion that if asked which I would prefer on my tombstone, "He was a very nice chap" or "He was a very good doctor", I would settle for the latter and leave it to my family and friends to remember me otherwise. Being nice to everyone is not always compatible with good doctoring, and perhaps another case will illustrate this point. I cannot remember precise details but a young boy of 14 or so was brought in by his mother for my advice. He was grossly obese and, as usual, "everything had been tried without success". I told him in no uncertain terms that he just had to stop eating so much and was later informed by his mother that her son "had never been so insulted" and had vowed never to see me again. I had forgotten the incident when about 25 years later a man in his late 30s brought his son in to see me. I didn't recognise him, but after the consultation he reminded me that he was the boy who had been so upset. He told me how angry he had been but then went on candidly to confess that it was the first time anyone had made him see that responsibility for his behaviour lay within himself. As a result he felt he had grown up, and took charge of his eating habits with beneficial results on his weight. Before he left the consultation room he told me that he had waited a long time to tell me this and was glad the opportunity had at last been afforded him.

In the late 70s, I found myself as a member of the medical services committee: this was the body that sat in judgment on general practitioners against whom complaints had been made. It consisted of a maximum of three professional members (doctors) and three lay members with a presiding chairman, who in our case was a practising solicitor. In theory the committee was composed of an equal number of doctors and lay members and if there was a split vote, the chairman had the casting vote. Usually two or three doctors found the time to attend but sometimes the lay members were short in numbers, in consequence of which the decision-making was rather lop-sided. If any question of behaviour by the doctor came to be questioned, the lay members would always ask the professionals if the behaviour was usual practice or not, and then accept their given opinion. I found it rather disconcerting sometimes when the question would be asked in the negative form. "Surely you wouldn't have behaved like that would you?" we were asked. Usually the answer of my colleagues would be, "Oh no, certainly not", but I knew that a more honest response would have been: "Sometimes, yes." Later this form of tribunal was abandoned as being too biased in favour of the doctor, but for some of us the scales went too far in the opposite direction. The common pattern became the lay people voting against the doctor and the professional members reacting to this by voting in favour, although in my experience when there were obvious and serious complaints, the professional members were quite strong in their condemnation of the doctor. On one occasion the case against the doctor was very flimsy, and unusually one of the lay members voted that there had been no breach. The chairman, who was not legally qualified, but someone who always gave me the impression that doctors were all as bad as each other and needed to be brought to book, seemed bereft without his casting vote. I heard him turn to another lay member and say, "We have lost that one." So much for the impartiality of the chairman.

I had for some time become disenchanted with the system of disciplining GPs and this episode was the last straw. I resigned from the committee and, in true gamekeeper-turned-poacher fashion, found myself acting as adviser and advocate for GPs summoned before the committee. This was much to the disgust of one chairman who felt this to be undemocratic and attempted to have me disbarred from acting for a doctor who had to appear before him. His objections were turned down, and I started a short but satisfying time as an advocate.

By the mid 1990s I felt I had enough experience of general practice and a basic knowledge of litigation and so decided I would move my area of interest into the field of expert witnessing. I was in the last few years before finally retiring from full time general practice, and I started my search for the best way to enter this new field. Clearly I needed a firmer base to my knowledge of legal procedures than mere experience had given me. To gain this I applied for, and was accepted to do, a course in arbitration. This was a short but intensive course organised by the Chartered Institute of Arbitrators, culminating in a short written exam, the passing of which bestowed the accolade of being an associate (ACIArb). The course was most rewarding and supplied the knowledge I was seeking. Of the 30 or so people on the course, I was the only medical doctor, most of the pupils being surveyors. I found the exam at the end of the course rather daunting and did not know what the expected pass rate was. I had not had to sit an exam for over 40 years, but the fluttering in my stomach when presented with the first paper brought back vivid memories of sitting finals as a young man. I was not altogether reassured when a friend, in an attempt to increase my confidence, asked if I had paid for the course. When I answered in the affirmative he cynically reassured me that "they always pass you if you've paid for the privilege of sitting the exam". I doubt very much the accuracy of his observation, but in the event I was relieved and pleased to be told that I had passed and could now add the letters ACIArb after my name. Later this was advanced to being a member, or MCIArb.

I was now au fait with the concept of how the level of proof in a civil case differed from that in a criminal case: "balance of probabilities" against "beyond reasonable doubt". I knew that balance of probabilities meant "more likely than not", or in practical terms, 51% of it being so: but I still remain troubled by the conflict this throws up when compared with the ethical responsibilities I have as a doctor. I am unlikely to persuade my legal colleagues that if they have only a 49% chance of treatment curing their disease, it is not worth treating them at all. I was also aware that my duty was firstly to the court and not to the solicitor or client who had instructed me and was paying my fees. It is worth commenting on the fact that until the Woolf reforms of the civil procedure rules in 1998, this was sometimes observed more in the breach than the action. The reforms highlighted this duty, and all expert witness reports now have to include a declaration to the court and a statement of truth, confirming one has acceded to this requirement.

At this time a new academic body had been founded, the Expert Witness Institute (EWI). As with the Institute of Arbitrators, I felt that membership would help highlight my credentials, but the next obstacle to becoming a recognised expert witness was a catch-22 situation: in order to become a member one had to supply references from two solicitors by whom one had been instructed. How to obtain these first two instructions is still one of the problems concerning new entrants. Since that time, the EWI have initiated an associate membership during which a mentor is provided to help and advise on any problems likely to be met in the early years as an expert. I was elected a fellow of the EWI in 2005, since when I have acted as mentor, but this particular catch 22 remains an obstacle that is hard to overcome.

Almost at the point of despair, I was fortunate to meet a colleague with whom I had previously worked in the department of general practice at St Bartholomew's. He was a young, bright Australian doctor who had returned to home base but was on a visit to the UK and we found ourselves visiting the department at the same time. My interest in medico-legal work and my difficulty in getting started somehow came in to the conversation, and he told me that while he had worked in England he had done a few cases for a firm of solicitors in the city, and he promised he would pass my name on to them. He did just that and my good fortune continued, as they had a case pending at that time. When they offered it to me I readily agreed. I remember it was around Christmas when I got all the papers and I spent much of the holiday reading a very large bundle of documents and writing up my report. I was delighted when they agreed to be a referee for my application to the EWI, and together with references from another solicitor with whom I had been associated and a High Court Judge known to me, I was admitted into membership and could now offer myself to other solicitors as an expert witness, my area of expertise being general practice. I have restricted myself nearly entirely to clinical negligence cases, and have avoided doing personal injury work. Work has drastically reduced since my CV has made it clear to potential instructing solicitors that I have reached an age – together with the added years it takes before a case is likely to come to court or fruition – when my expertise of the here-and-now may be called into question by cross-examining barristers. During the 15 years I have been involved as an expert witness, I have written over 300 reports, but only been called upon to attend court on about a dozen occasions. I have mostly been instructed by solicitors acting on behalf of claimants, but about a quarter of the cases were instructed by the defendant. I was also involved in a dispute between GP partners, having been instructed by the court as a single joint expert.

I have found the work stimulating and interesting. There have been downsides, mainly when a case in which you have convinced yourself you are correct in the opinion you have given, but which the court (by which I mean the judge) finds against the client who has instructed you to write the report. Settling of fees within a reasonable time sometimes proved difficult, but I was always paid in the end.

Frequently, I have heard it said that an expert could only be relevant if he or she is in active practice. I disagree with this: in my experience, I have found that it was only in the early years of retirement that I found the time needed to fully inspect and analyse the bundle of documents, which often amounted to several hundred pages. Reports from experts who are in full time practice, can easily miss an important fact hidden deep inside the bundle, but which are of vital importance to the case.

I have now retired completely from offering my services as an expert witness, having accepted that the period since being in active practice, and the numerous changes that have been made in the way that medicine is now practiced, has become a bar to my being able to offer the standard of expertise that a client should expect. Although this is a cause of regret, I must record that my experiences of the legal system in Great Britain has left me with some reservations as to its fairness in reaching a result. The so-called adversarial system troubles me; a decision tends to be settled by whoever has argued the case better rather than by a fair assessment of all the facts. Lawyers have cocooned themselves from any responsibility that a miscarriage of justice may have occurred by rules of procedure. These factors have led to a tendency for cross examination to be aggressive, and judges tending towards omnipotence. The inquisitorial system (as practiced in many other countries) has many weaknesses, but a combination of the two, I feel, might lead to a fairer form of justice than we have at present.

CHAPTER XXI

Fundholding

In my time, successive governments have repeatedly tried to introduce cost-saving elements to the NHS, doing so under the euphemistic title of reform. I don't think it can be denied that the professions working in the NHS have grown weary of trying to keep up with what the politicians have tried to impose upon them after the latest results from focus groups (another euphemism, they would be better called pressure groups). However, and on looking back on the changes that have occurred as a result of many of these reforms, and with the benefit of hindsight, I now believe that there has been some overall improvement in the management of primary care to the advantage of patients, but not without frustration to those working within the NHS.

From the birth of the NHS in 1948 until the 1970s, very little changed within primary care other than the improvements being seen as a result of the efforts of the general practitioners themselves. It was Sir Keith Joseph, secretary of state for health in the Thatcher government, who first introduced a revolutionary change or reform, in which management was divided between district management teams (DMTs, responsible for co-ordinated health care of the locality), area management teams (AMTs, responsible for a group of localities), and regional management teams (RMTs, responsible for the whole region). Although in theory these teams had no hierarchical structure, inevitably, in practice, each knew its place and deferred to the team above them. Anyone working within one of these teams (as I did in a DMT) was aware of this underlying truth. Notwithstanding this, the system did have definite advantages. In the first place it reunited to a certain extent, and for the first time, the three elements of primary care, hospital services and public health. It also allowed primary care to have some say in how the local services were managed by introducing a compulsory representative from general practice as a member of the team. Another consequence of this arrangement was that public health, working as they did from base headquarters, inevitably became more powerful in decision making. It was also decreed that the GP and consultant members of the team alternated as chairman, which allowed discussion, but not necessarily implementation, of what was considered important in primary care. I had been nominated by the local medical committee to be the GP representative, and I think had some success in altering the fixed views of the previous hospital management committees, who were completely blinkered to our needs. (The "good GP", in the view of too many consultants, bore no resemblance to his abilities as a clinician, but more to whether he was willing to carry out the consultant's orders with no questions asked, and also to look after any emergencies that might occur in the absence of the consultant.) On the down side of this arrangement, it was clear to me that when the GP was acting as chairman of the Team and trying to discuss problems within primary care, the consultant member often stayed away.

Fundholding was introduced in 1991 by the then-secretary of state Kenneth Clarke, a jovial and good-humoured man with an underlying rottweiler instinct and a strong belief that the medical profession were out only for themselves and could only be humanised by the promise of money. These were ideas reminiscent of his predecessor and the implementer of the NHS, Aneurin Bevan. GPs, on the other hand, felt left behind in the financial benefits due to them, from the hard studying and heavy workload in which they were involved. I think many of us felt that making more money was not immoral, but still wanted to contribute fully to working within the health service.

Perhaps because it was being imposed upon the profession, fundholding had to face up to strong opposition and eventually was killed off by a Labour government coming to power and wanting to undo anything that had been put in place by the previous Conservative government (at least as far as the health service was concerned). Hospital doctors opposed it because they perceived they would lose some, if not all, the power they held in controlling NHS funding. Many GPs were concerned that they had enough on their plate and felt that the added responsibility of managing their practices would overwhelm them. Some were against it on political grounds; it was not the policy of the party they supported so they would not help it flourish. (Interestingly, in recent years the Labour party has tried to re-introduce what is fundholding in all but name, under the new term "commissioning".) The British Medical Association (BMA) came out against it for no reason that I could fathom, other than that its hospital doctor membership was very much larger than its GP membership. On the whole the media, if not entirely against the idea, certainly did not support it. The Royal College of General Practitioners sat on the fence so firmly they could never see their way to saying yea or nay until it was much too late. Other observers thought the idea good but were concerned it may give too much power to GPs. I discussed the matter with many colleagues and eventually came to the conclusion that, properly run, it could be the pot of gold at the end of the rainbow for which we had all been searching for a long time.

I was not a novice to the idea of making the most of rules and regulations in a bid to improve the level of service we could offer our patients. Having joined a single handed practitioner nearing retirement due to ill health in 1957, and having seen the practice grow with the help of a new breed of incoming partners to a six partner group practice by the time I retired in 1998, I was not unaware of how to improve services and eventually receive financial help to put these improvements into practice. My first venture into this sphere was in 1959 when I managed to persuade the then medical officer of health (MOH) for Hackney, to let us have an attached health visitor for the baby clinic we wanted to run on a regular basis within the practice. According to my research (although I am prepared for this to be disputed) I was only the second GP in London to actually have a health visitor present at a baby clinic. (In spite of the commendable forward vision of Dr King, the MOH in question, it took another 25 to 30 years before we could persuade Hackney that a full time health visitor attachment to the practice would be beneficial to the patients. It was quite amazing how what had seemed an impossibility for so many years was transformed, almost over-night, by a single forward-looking senior nursing officer who recognised the need for it and set it in motion.)

For many years I had found that if an improvement to the running of the practice or the care of the patients had been shown to be feasible by other innovative GPs in the country, there was no point in waiting for a new government reform (that word again) to fund it. Supplying one's own funding from income was the only way to make it happen. Over the years I found that the biggest increase to practice income came from official recognition that a particular service was necessary, and full or partial reimbursement would be paid by the NHS for a service that previously the practice had been funding. This happened with the employing of reception and secretarial staff, paying for an attached practice nurse, and improving the practice premises. We had benefited from all these innovations, but the final outcome was that the practice was funded in a very random fashion. We had ancillary staff (nurse, practice manager, secretary and receptionists) who we paid and were reimbursed up to 70% (the 30% we were left to pay was, by this time, a considerable slice out of the gross income for the prac-tice): we also had attached staff (practice nurses and a health visi-tor) who were paid by the NHS, but also employed by them and it was, therefore, outside our control to appoint them or influence their terms of service. Finally we also had an attached counsellor for whom we were not reimbursed. A counsellor had attended the practice since the early 1970s. At that time they were marriage guidance counsellors, and had agreed to attend on a purely volun-tary and unpaid basis and for many years gave sterling service. Later their role was extended to provide general counselling and they were paid for the service. I could see that the first benefit of fundholding would be that all these random services could come together and be paid for out of a budget controlled by us.

I think we were right, even if rather arrogant, in our belief that this would improve the service to the patients. One fundamental change created by fundholding was that the GP would negotiate a budget for all the services he provided out of which he would be responsible for paying the bills (with some exceptions, in order to ensure certain basic services, such as the ambulance service, were not interfered with.) At first, and presumably in order to encourage GPs to accept the principle, any surplus made between the budget agreed and the total spent could be kept by the GP. This caused such a roar of disapproval that it was rapidly changed to a percentage of the savings that had to be used for agreed improvements to practice care. The term "budget practices" was rapidly changed to "fundholding practices", a term that remained in use.

Having seen the benefit of fundholding both to the way we ran our practice and to the way we perceived we could improve the services we were supplying, it took very little time for my partners to agree we should apply to become "first-wave" fundholders. It was also agreed that I would be the practice fundholder leader in the discussions with the health authorities that were fundamental to the scheme. This was 1991, and as far as I was concerned, a new lease of life and enthusiasm became part of the remaining years I had in practice before retiring in 1998.

On judging the phases of my professional life, I think I can safely say that there were three elements that contributed to my having a successful and emotionally fulfilling time in general practice. Firstly, general practice, I am sure, was the correct branch of medicine for me; and the good fortune I had in the choice of partners over the years added to the satisfaction with which I can look back. Secondly, the years I spent teaching at both undergraduate and postgraduate levels were important; my only regret now is that I did not record the names of all those with whom I became involved so that I would now know what had become of them.

Finally I must point to the eight or nine years in which we were fundholders: for us it created the way forward to practice at the standards we had set ourselves, and it provided great emotional satisfaction as well as, I hope, vastly improved services to our patients.

Having made the decision to be fundholders, and having been accepted as such by the health authority, the next task was to oversee it's setting up in the practice. Regular meetings, usually at weekly intervals, were held with the partners and practice manager and occasional meetings were also held with the area health authority and other suppliers, including the private sector, to discuss details of commissioning. Perhaps the most important element of fundholding that helped it to be successful was the acceptance by the government that if the scheme was to succeed practices would need a management allowance to run it. This was included in the overall budget that was negotiated with the health authority. At the time, many voices spoke out against the idea, thinking it a waste of public money, but the percentage of the overall cost was never more than 2% to 3% of the total budget.

We suspected that most people working within the NHS had very little idea of running a business – indeed this, in my opinion, remains one of the fundamental problems in trying to run a financially feasible health service. We decided, therefore, to look to the business world to find a business manager to run the fundholding element, while the practice manager continued to be responsible for the day-to-day running of the practice. Many other practices decided to combine the duties of practice manager with budget manager which, in my opinion, was not always successful.

We were fortunate to appoint an accountant who had spent many years of his working life in senior management with one of the largest retail stores in the country. He had recently retired, but was still young enough to look for part-time work, and readily agreed to join us in our venture. Although his knowledge of how the health service worked was not great, he soon learned:

of greater importance he introduced a business element to the running of this new behemoth with which we were struggling. As a result of his expertise we were able to negotiate a satisfactory budget that allowed us to carry out many innovations that had previously been impossible. We could now employ our own practice nurses rather than rely on the local authority supplying them "when available". Marriage guidance on a voluntary basis could now be extended to full counselling services, a move that saved many patients from the need to be referred to hospital for a psychiatric opinion. Patients' wishes to receive treatment from complementary practitioners were partially satisfied by employing an acupuncturist, though we drew the line at some other therapies for which there was no evidence of benefit.

A natural extension to these additional services being provided within the practice premises was to organise consultants to attend the surgery to see patients rather than patients having to attend hospital for the privilege. A gynaecologist, an ear, nose and throat (ENT) surgeon, a psychiatrist, a dermatologist and a rheumatologist all provided in-house clinics, almost making long waiting lists a thing of the past. A variation of this system became necessary when the ENT surgeon found he could no longer attend in person: we arranged for a reserved number of appointments that we could make directly from the practice for the patient to attend at hospital. I believe this system is being encouraged at the present time. One reason for the very long waiting lists at some clinics became clear when I discussed with a local consultant dermatologist the possibility of reserving a few appointments for our practice, which we would pay for, but give back for general use if they had not been taken up by a reasonable time before they were due. He explained that his problem with appointments was that he had to accept every GP referral, but there was one local single-handed GP who regularly took up a third to a half of all his appointments, mostly with patients that could have very well been treated by the GP himself. Another example of the impotence of the system to improve the standards of care, was the problem that obstetricians were having with a minority of GPs who were being paid to provide shared care, but who were not even bothering to provide the antenatal care that was so essential to avoid complications in pregnancy. I suggested that since they had to give permission for the GP to share the care before he or she could be paid, they should withdraw that permission if they did not feel the practitioner was providing a satisfactory service. For some reason they did not feel this was possible.

Without going too far into the rather complicated subject of how the NHS funded health care within the hospital service, it is worth recording another incongruity that bedevilled financing and which was exposed, I think, by fundholding. Most services provided by hospitals were paid for on the basis that they were given a budget that was supposed to cover all the services they provided, a so-called block budget. Inevitably this led to a conflict for available resources, with the more powerful hospitals getting the lion's share from central management, and within the hospital itself the more powerful practitioners creaming off the majority portion. "Cinderella services" such as mental health and geriatrics were left way behind and the same problems exist to this day. Payment, in the main, was made as a block payment and the hospital would then deal with whatever was sent to them. This did not suit us in fundholding practices since we wanted greater control of our finances. An alternative type of contract that we could negotiate was the cost-per-service contract. We would pay the price of the procedure when it was needed. The first problem to overcome was to find out how much each individual procedure actually cost. This was heavily resisted by the hospitals since they had never had to work this out under the block contract system. For the first time, the importance of how much a procedure actually cost – and could be sold for – became apparent. Some interesting figures emerged, an example of which may give an insight into how the system was flawed. When hospitals were finally persuaded to give figures, we were informed by two different teaching hospitals that the cost of a particular gynaecological procedure (on an admittedly very rare complaint) was either £3,000 by one hospital or £6,000 by the other. It was quite obvious that should one of our patients require the procedure, it would be common sense, if facilities were equally satisfactory, to send her to the cheaper hospital. (It must be said here that other procedures were more expensive at the "cheaper" hospital, so the system was really quite random.) Curiosity persuaded me to research this difference in price and the conclusion I reached was that both hospitals only knew the total cost for all gynaecological services and neither knew the price for the individual procedure. They had, therefore, divided the total expenditure by the number of cases they had treated to arrive at the figure. One hospital had only treated one case that year and the other had treated two, thus appearing to have spent only half the amount of the more expensive provider.

*

The criticisms of fundholding were, in my opinion, unfair and were largely responsible for the demise of a system that might have avoided the difficulties the NHS now finds itself in. "Two-tier system" is the cry that always seems to spring up when anything is attempted that is perceived to be too expensive. Of course, in the early days, those of us who had opted to accept fundholding were in a better position to improve services to our patients than those who opted to stay out of it. This is how all beneficial innovations start, but eventually those that prove helpful come into general use, and the improvements become established practice. After we were up and running in our practice I had no qualms in reporting that with fundholding, if adequately funded and properly run, private practice would no longer be necessary. Another cry from the "anti" brigade was that fundholding introduced the market into medicine, where it had no place. If by market is meant that it brought to light how services were actually financed, then I would not argue, but surely this would have been of benefit, especially to those services that the hospital sector judged to be unimportant, but which GPs recognised as representing a majority of the needs of the population.

A final nail hammered into the coffin of fundholding was the belief that it was too generous to some doctors. At the beginning there was some truth in this assertion, but as time passed and everyone became more aware of the pitfalls and true costs, budgets were adjusted; in any case any money saved by prudent housekeeping was ploughed back into the practice for the benefit of the patients.

By the time I retired in 1998, fundholding had been given its death notice: although not greatly mourned at the time, I hope this chapter about it will at least act as a memorial to what I believe was a lost opportunity.

CHAPTER XXII

Abortion

The word abortion is often used pejoratively, but in fact it should, more accurately, be defined as both spontaneous abortion (better known as a miscarriage) and induced abortion (a termination of pregnancy). It is within the latter meaning that there is such a wide spectrum of feeling, ranging from complete prohibition under any circumstances to abortion-on-demand. The abortion act of 1967 in this country tried to establish a compromise, allowing termination of pregnancy under certain conditions, but maintaining the illegality of "on-demand". Probably because of the wide disparity of views that still exists, the issue remains to this day highly contentious, with politicians and pressure groups each espousing their own views and, some might say, leaving the woman with an unwanted pregnancy in the middle. Inevitably, in these circumstances, the general practitioner, who remains the doctor of first contact for most patients, and the gynaecologist, who has to carry out the procedure, are left in the front line of decision-making. The rest of the population has the luxury of only having a theoretical problem to solve.

In the 1950s and early 1960s induced abortion was illegal except under rigid circumstances such as the health of the mother being at greater risk if the pregnancy was allowed to continue: this was usually interpreted as "serious health risk" or even as "risk to the life of the mother". In some ways this made decision-making for the GP, when faced with a difficult case, much easier. One could only offer sympathy and what woefully inadequate help was available, often in the form of charitable but rather inhospitable homes, which would look after the expectant mother in the later weeks or months of pregnancy, before the baby would be taken away for adoption. This was an improvement, perhaps, on the

189

workhouses of the 19th century, but not a very happy solution for any woman finding herself in this predicament. It is only very recently that the all too frequent cruel consequences to both mother and child of this regime has been exposed.

In the years after the passing of the abortion act it became easier to refer women for whom termination was deemed to be appropriate, but there were still ambivalent feelings among GPs and gynaecologists. Both varied in their views on the appropriateness of termination, rationalised to themselves as being ethical or non-ethical, but in reality depending on their own emotional feelings and needs. A woman with an unwanted pregnancy had to be careful to choose a GP known to be sympathetic to her condition, and the GP, in turn, had to know where he could refer her with any hope that the termination would be carried out. Artificial standards were created in an attempt to keep the rising demand under some control. For instance, some doctors rigorously maintained the same high standards of what constituted increased risk to the health of the woman prior to the act, while some would put a limit to the period of gestation before they would consider carrying out the procedure. A woman who was more than 14 weeks pregnant might find her request refused on the grounds that termination would involve invasive surgery (a hysterotomy) which carried a greater risk than the less invasive D and C (dilatation and curettage) or suction curettage which were the methods used up to about 12-weeks gestation. The tricky situation that ensued was that with the enormous demands on the NHS, gynaecological waiting lists were long enough to push the woman beyond 12 or 14 weeks before she was even seen by the gynaecologist, even if the referral had been made in plenty of time. Not surprisingly, the private sector, if it was prepared to be involved in terminations, flourished and in some areas (possibly the majority) the only way to have a termination was through the private sector, making it financially prohibitive to a large number of women.

An additional problem was the perennial misuse by the population of failing to differentiate between needs and wants. I am sure I am not alone in the belief that if the distinction between needs and wants had been clarified and enforced at the start of the health service, it might be in a better position to cope with its financial difficulties today. No society, whether global, international, national or local, can afford to finance all the wants of its population, but in many cases it might be possible to cope with the needs. A late attempt by the government to introduce a controlling body, the National Institute for Clinical Evidence, or NICE, to keep the costs of treatment within reasonable boundaries, has proved to be very unpopular when their judgment of what constitutes need (measured rather ambivalently in terms of quality of life) is called into question.

Not surprisingly, given the demand for termination but lack of facilities to provide it to all for whom it was requested, together with the relative shortage of doctors sympathetic enough to be helpful, the health service facilities were gradually supplanted by the private sector. An additional service also flourished in response to the need: the termination clinics. Often these were extensions and additions to the family-planning clinics that were already providing contraceptive advice, either with or without referral from the GP. Their philosophy was very well summed up in an advertisement to the public that stated: "Pregnant and happy – fine, but if not, contact us . . ." Their presence meant quicker and earlier referral for those finding themselves with an unwanted pregnancy, but they were also, at least partially, responsible for the lowering of the standard of the indications that were (and are) still necessary for the procedure to be legal within the act. Although counselling was offered, this was too often acknowledged "mainly in the breach". The distinction between termination on medical grounds and abortion-on-demand became more and more blurred; the debate continues to this day.

So far I have discussed the universal aspect of some of the problems involved, but I have not said very much about my own experiences. I have no religious or deeply felt moral objections to the procedure, and believe that a woman does have the right to chose, but perhaps too often is given this freedom without accepting the responsibility that goes with it. The GP is often in the position of being mediator rather than arbitrator when consulted by a woman who feels she cannot face up to continuation of her pregnancy. I have recognised in myself that when a woman has been undecided about her emotional and physical needs, I have felt more fulfilled if she decides on continuation rather than termination and perhaps this may have created some bias in my counselling. Being able to hide behind the illegality of the procedure made it easier, but it may not always have resulted in the most appropriate outcome. In about 1960 I remember being consulted by a patient who was about the same age as me. She came with her husband, and I knew the family quite well. They had three children from about the age of six upwards. She had become pregnant unexpectedly, probably because of contraceptive failure. The thought of a fourth child was impossible to contemplate, on both financial and emotional grounds. At the time, termination was not an option unless there were clear-cut medical reasons, and these were difficult to find. However, she made it quite clear that she knew exactly where to go and how to obtain an abortion if it was not available under the NHS. We discussed the matter at some length and finally she and her husband decided that they would go through with the pregnancy and somehow cope. At the time I was unaware to what extent I might have influenced their decision, but looking back on it now, recognition of my own feelings towards termination and the fact that both myself and my wife are fourth children (who in similar circumstances might not be here) must have played some part, even if I was unaware of it. All seemed to be well, and both parents appeared happy at the prospect of another child, when late in pregnancy (and much too late to do anything about it) not even twins, but triplets were diagnosed. All of them were born healthy and although outwardly they remained happy-looking, I am still unsure whether the looks they gave me were full of reproach or not . . . I was reminded of the great Shakespearean lines from *Twelfth Night*: "Some are born great, some achieve greatness and some have greatness thrust upon them!"

The increasing availability of contraception at the time in question created an additional problem. The contraceptive pill became available around the same time that the abortion act was passed, and soon after the intrauterine device (IUD). Prior to this, and at a time when termination was not available legally to most pregnant women, preventing pregnancy was achieved by the following, often not too reliable methods: condoms worn by men; dutch caps, or similar, worn by women; withdrawal prior to climax (*coitus interruptus*), used commonly, I am informed, in some countries in Europe, but not too often in this country; the "safe period", which involved keeping count of the days within a woman's menstrual cycle during which it was deemed to be safe to have intercourse without becoming pregnant; and abstention, a method not very popular with most young people except, perhaps, on religious grounds. Another method was the so-called Graffenberg ring, named after its inventor. This was already going out of fashion by the time I qualified, and wasn't a contraceptive at all, but a device that caused bleeding which would have to be investigated. This involved a D and C that in turn caused any possible pregnancy to be terminated. It was, in fact, a device by which abortion could be carried out legally.

In the late 1950s I was asked by a colleague to act as a locum for his private patients while he was away on holiday for three weeks. I was pleased to accept, the extra money bringing some welcome relief to what were still hard times. Not surprisingly there was very little to do, most patients preferring to wait and see their own doctor unless the condition was urgent. Rather to my surprise a lady in her late 40s approached me: she had two grown up children and was very concerned at having become pregnant unintentionally. In this case, her psychological state was such that I had no qualms at being able to agree that termination was not only justified, but also medically essential. However, examination revealed her to be about the size of a 16-week gestation – that is, the womb extended into the abdomen and had reached the height halfway between the rim of the pelvis and the umbilicus. An open hysterotomy would be required, and as at the time I held a part-time position as a clinical assistant in gynaecology at the local hospital, I turned to the consultant with whom I worked for advice and help. We agreed that a domiciliary visit at her home would be appropriate and arrangements were made for us to meet there. He confirmed my findings on examination and agreed that termination was necessary. Arrangements were made for her to be admitted the next day for the procedure to be carried out, and as was not unusual at that time, he agreed to me acting as his assistant at the operation. The time for operation approached and we were all scrubbed up; the anaesthetist had carried out his job and our patient had been wheeled into the operating theatre and lifted on to the table. As her outer robe was removed there was a gasp as it became immediately noticeable that her stomach was as flat as a pancake! Where had her 16-week pregnancy gone? A vaginal examination by the gynaecologist confirmed a normal sized uterus and the diagnosis became clear. It was a perfect case of so-called pseudocyesis or false pregnancy. This condition is well documented but, in such floridity, rarely encountered. The lump had been caused by unconscious tightening of her abdominal muscles into a perfect shape of a 16-week uterus, and the relaxation caused as she became unconscious from the anaesthetic, flattened her abdominal wall like a balloon losing its gas. Fortunately, rather than thinking of suing us for an incorrect diagnosis, our patient was delighted both at not being pregnant and the care she had received. A rather unhappy sequel to the affair occurred about two weeks later. My wife received a call from her husband to say that he would like to thank me for the care his wife had received, and as he was a dress manufacturer, he would like to send one of his vans to our flat with some dresses from which she could choose one she liked. That same afternoon a delivery van full of dresses was parked in the driveway, and the driver brought up to the flat three dresses from which she could chose. Unfortunately, he had forgotten to lock the van and by the time he had returned to it, it had been stolen, together with half his stock of dresses that were in the process of being delivered to the retail shops.

It did not take long after the abortion act was passed for the "sharks" to move in, in an attempt to fill their own pockets. It was at this time that I became aware of a scheme devised to profit from other people's misfortunes. The area in which I practiced had several cab drivers among the residents, some of whom were my patients. The vast majority lived honest and worthy lives, but among their number were some intent on increasing their income by whatever means possible, and for which abortion provided a great opportunity. One such cabbie, who was not my patient but informed me he had been recommended to speak to me by one, asked if I would meet some colleagues of his to discuss the setting up of a co-operative of drivers, for whom they needed a medical adviser. This fed my curiosity to the extent of agreeing to a meeting, which took place at an office in Kings Cross. It took only a few minutes to realise that my joining the scheme involved two important facts. First, I would earn a great deal of money and secondly any ideas of medical and personal ethics and morals that I possessed would fly out of the window. I knew at that moment that of the two, my personal integrity was of greater importance, but curiosity led me to play along a little longer in order to find out what was involved. As it later became public knowledge, I am not divulging any secrets when I explain what was involved. As abortion had now become legal in this country, but was still illegal in many countries elsewhere, particularly in Ireland, an agency was being set up to ship pregnant women to Britain, where they would be accommodated for three to five days and during which time they would undergo termination of their unwanted pregnancy. They would then be returned home and all this for one overall fee. The involved taxi drivers would act as the couriers and agents, retaining an agency fee for themselves. The only remaining elements for the scheme to work was to find doctors willing to carry out the terminations and sign the necessary certificates with no questions asked in order to make it legal. My function would have been to provide the second signature for which I would be paid by the taxi driver acting as agent. The relief I felt at getting out of the office is difficult to describe, especially as I realised that if some form of mafia was not already involved, one very soon would be. Soon after this, phone booths were full of notices of numbers that could be used by pregnant women wanting an abortion with no strings attached, as long as they had the money to pay.

By the late 1970s, experience and my own views had crystallised my attitude to abortion into being sympathetic to the requests received, providing advice or counselling (and the two are not the same thing) is given and the woman is fully informed. I have no doubt my own prejudices and biases may have coloured my actions from time to time, but I hope I have been, at least, partly successful.

CHAPTER XXIII

Is There a Doctor in the House?

In the minds of many of the lay public the familiar cry of "Is there a doctor in the house?" is an every day occurrence during most doctors' lives. In reality, it is only rarely heard, and when it is it is greeted with a mixture of curiosity and anxiety that one may not be up to the unknown hazards that await. It is assumed that when the cry is heard, any doctor within earshot immediately downs tools and prepares himself for the task ahead of saving life and limb. Perhaps in an attempt to disabuse the embryo doctor, it was early on in our medical school training that we were told to remember that "the wise doctor runs for only two things – haemorrhage and nylon stockings". (At the time nylon stockings were in very short supply). In my experience I only heard the cry on rare occasions, perhaps every 10 years or so. Even so, in spite of the medical school advice, any reluctance to answer the call in case I found myself in a situation way out of my depth, would be quickly dissipated if anyone, not a doctor, was close by: the duty owed to society at large made it imperative that the call was answered, whatever the inconvenience, and added to the feelings of curiosity and anxiety would be a powerful foreboding that one's inadequacies were soon to be shown up.

The first occasion that I experienced these feelings was not related to "is there any doctor in the house", but to me personally as the newly appointed house doctor on my first day as a qualified doctor doing a house job at the London Hospital. The first day of my new job was a Sunday and we were all sitting at the lunch table enjoying roast lamb with all the trimmings. (In those days even busy young doctors were treated as "officer material" and not expected to slum it in the general hospital canteen.) Hardly had I started to enjoy the meal when a message came across the tannoy. "Doctor Carne to ring the ward immediately." An obvious emergency: it was the reason why I had spent the past seven years studying medicine; now theory was to be translated into practice; an interested observer was to become a responsible participant; instead of the luxury of asking questions, I was to have the responsibility of answering them. All eyes were on me as I picked up the phone attached to the wall in order to ring the designated ward. Everyone was curious as to what the nature of the emergency might be, and how I might cope. I dialled the number of the ward, and almost immediately the other end answered, "Staff nurse speaking, is that Doctor Carne?" Trying to convey the confidence I was a long way from feeling, I spoke rather more gruffly than I might have done. "Doctor Carne here, how can I help you?" (Please God, let it be straightforward was my unexpressed thought.) The reply rather staggered me. "While taking the temperature of a child," the staff nurse said, "he bit the thermometer in half and has swallowed the mercury contained in it. What should we do?" Seven years studying and not once had this happened to me or ever come to my attention. I repressed the desire to respond "How the hell should I know" and biding for time, which I hoped would give me a chance to find an answer that even if not professionally correct, might do no harm, I replied, somewhat less confidently, "I'll come up straight away."

Turning to my colleagues round the table, I was somewhat disturbed that they appeared to have lost all interest and had returned to eating their meal. "Does anyone know what to do for a child who has swallowed the contents of a bitten thermometer?" I asked in an attempt to restore their interest. At first no one answered or only expressed ignorance if they did. Then a lone voice came to my rescue: "I read somewhere that a cotton wool sandwich was the first aid treatment for swallowing glass; perhaps it may also absorb the mercury and then be passed out at the other end. At the very least, it may prevent any shafts of glass from the broken thermometer doing internal damage." Experience had not yet taught me that sometimes "masterly inactivity" is the most appropriate action of all, so I made my way to the ward feeling that at least I could advise the nursing staff to do something that they had not thought of and thus maintain the hierarchy between us. In the end, fortunately, the child came to no harm, but I was reminded of the incident many years later when a mercury thermometer I was carrying in my pocket on holiday was confiscated by a security guard at the airport on the basis that if it broke in flight, it could spread along the cabin and only a minute quantity might be sufficient to interfere with the mechanics of the plane and cause it to crash. If the contents of one thermometer can kill over 200 people, what harm might it have done to one single child?

One evening we were at the theatre with friends: I do not remember the name of the play, but during the interval our friends came running over to us to relay a message that I had pretended not to hear. There was an announcement asking if there was a doctor in the house. Trapped, I had no alternative but to retreat to the back of the theatre and make myself known to a very flustered front-of-house manager tending an elderly lady who was sitting in the now emptied bar, clutching her chest, and looking very pale. Even without the benefit of my medical gear (no doctor should be without it) I recognised that this was most probably a cardiac emergency. With some relief I was informed that an ambulance had been summoned and all I could do in the circumstances was to stay with the patient until it arrived. It was with some impatience I heard the three rings, followed a few minutes later by two rings and then after a further short interval one ring, telling the audience to return to their seats. With some consternation I viewed every one leaving the area and finally was left only with the individual who was now my patient and the manager who was now her guardian, making sure I did not leave her alone. The main topic of conversation was me reassuring the patient that all would be well and she would be in good hands at the hospital, and the manager reassuring her that he would give her tickets to return to the theatre to see the rest of the play once she was well. By the time the ambulance arrived and she was transferred into the capable hands of the paramedics, the second act of the play was well under way. Hoping I would be able to pick up what I had missed, I turned to the manager and asked to be escorted back to my seat. He said, "Oh, I can't let you in during the action; you will just have to stand at the back." No suggestion of compensation or, like the victim, seats for a future performance. It was just assumed I had done my duty and the matter was now closed. I never did discover how the play ended.

In the 1960s, licensed gambling casinos made their appearance in this country, and in the early days vied with each other to attract custom. Although they relied on the big spenders, they were quite keen to accommodate smaller players, and if you had a profession they felt you added extra cachet and were happy to let you play for quite small amounts but still give you the freebies used to attract custom. Fine dining at minimal cost was one of the benefits, although you had to be a bigger roller than I was to get it free. One of the more prestigious casinos was Crockfords, which had been associated with upper class gambling for at least two hundred years. Gambling there might be equated with watching horse racing from the royal enclosure at Ascot.

Of the various games played, I found roulette utterly boring, *chemin-de-feur* far too expensive and blackjack heart breaking. However, one game which had been exported from America was dice, or craps. Not only are the odds quite good if you play it correctly, but it is fast, noisy and exciting. In addition you were your own master, rather than having a croupier acting for you. I watched other people play and learned the rules and the odds you could obtain and eventually graduated to playing, but as was inevitable with the bad luck that I always attract when I gamble, rarely had the excitement of a winning streak. I'm told, when it happens, you feel as if you rule the world and anything is possible. I nearly reached this apotheosis one night when I found myself rolling the dice, and things were going my way. I had achieved four winning throws in a row and in my euphoric state expected to achieve many more; then out of the corner of my eye I caught sight of an elderly gentleman sitting on a couch behind me, holding his chest and becoming more and more ashen faced. Duty kept tugging at me to see if he needed my assistance, but gambling greed, like a devil on my shoulder, kept whispering in my ear: "You may never have such an opportunity again!" I had one more throw, which continued my successful streak, but then noted he was looking even worse, and I returned to my senses. Reluctantly I passed the dice to my neighbour, much to the annoyance of all the other players who were benefiting from my successful roll of the dice, and turned to the troubled gentleman, who by now was surrounded by the manager, the pit boss and several curious customers, but no doctors among them. Once again it was obvious that the most likely cause of his symptoms arose in his heart, and transfer to a hospital as quickly as possible was essential. He had probably never experienced care from the NHS in his life, but this was an emergency when a blue-light ambulance and local hospital was the obvious course of action to be taken. Ignoring his requests, rapidly turning into demands, that he be transferred to a private hospital, I eventually succeeded in convincing him that on a Saturday night the large teaching hospital within a mile of the casino was really the best option. I also assured him that I would accompany him to the hospital and make sure he was treated immediately and appropriately. I managed to get him seen quickly and tests confirmed he had had a heart attack; appropriate treatment was given. After about an hour he was safely tucked up in bed and I left to return to the casino, by which time any positive thoughts of continuing my lucky streak had disappeared. I collected my wife and we returned home.

It later transpired that the gentleman I had escorted to hospital was a privileged member of Crockfords and in recognition of my actions the casino, showing greater generosity than the theatre manager, offered me honorary life-time membership of the club – worth quite a lot of money. Unfortunately the bad luck I attracted as a gambler continued, and after I had used the membership a couple of times, ownership of the casino changed hands. After a period of closure, Crockfords reopened under new management who did not renew my honorary membership. This may have been a blessing in disguise: I gave up going to casinos altogether.

One hot, midsummer day I was enjoying a day at the cricket at Lords. I had managed to obtain a ticket for the test match between England and Australia, and the languid day was interrupted by an announcement over the loudspeakers asking if there was a doctor among the spectators, and if so would they please go to the pavilion. As there was no one with me to expose my identity, I slid lower in the seat and hoped I would not be noticed. About ten minutes later the plea for a doctor was repeated. This time I thought there might be a secondary gain in answering the call; meeting international cricketers would fulfil a boyhood ambition and might prove ample reward for such a minor interruption. I might, I fantasised, even be instrumental in saving England from defeat. The healing hand on the injured or sick English player might be enough to allow him to return to the field of conflict, where his presence would transfer an inevitable defeat into a sterling victory. I made my way round the outskirts of the ground towards the pavilion and when I arrived, said to the steward standing in front of the gate like a guard on sentry duty: "I understand you are in need of a doctor." I waited for his face to show a sign of relief and for the gates to be opened to allow me to enter the holy of holies, but all I got was a smile, almost of contempt, and a finger pointing to the 'nursery end' as he said: "Yes sir. Just join the queue over there please . . ." I slunk back to my seat and enjoyed the rest of the day's cricket.

Returning by airplane from a holiday in the Far East, I was awoken by one of the cabin staff asking if I was a medical doctor. On answering yes he apologised for disturbing me but requested that I have a look at a passenger who appeared to have been taken ill. Apparently a gentleman in the seat behind me had ordered a cup of coffee, at which time he appeared to be quite well, but on lifting the cup to his mouth he spilt it all over himself, and complained of a non-functioning left arm and hand. He was conscious and able to speak, and the diagnosis was obviously a stroke, but the extent of it was unclear. I was travelling with my brother-in-law, also a doctor, and on the basis of two heads being better than one, I asked him to join in the consultation. There was little we could do but observe him, especially as the emergency medical box carried by the plane, although full of defibrillators and cardiograph machines, had no simple aspirin, which might have been useful as a first-aid drug in the circumstances.

The captain of the flight, when informed, was concerned as to whether he should return to Singapore, about three hours flight away, land at the nearest airport, which I think was somewhere in India, or carry on the flight to London Heathrow. Half an hour's observation confirmed our patient was not deteriorating, remained compos mentis but was still hemiplegic. Both doctors agreed that we should advise continuing the flight but be prepared to land if our patient's condition showed signs of worsening. Heathrow should be warned to have an ambulance standing by so he could be transferred to hospital immediately on landing. Overnight we kept an eye on him and remained reassured that he showed no signs of deterioration; we managed to reach Heathrow without further incident. Problems did arise, however, after we landed. Firstly the ambulance had not been ordered as we believed and we had to wait about an hour for one to arrive. Meanwhile all the other passengers and most of the crew left the plane while we dutifully remained with our patient in case he came to harm. The next problem was when the ambulance arrived with the stretcher party to take the stricken man off the plane. We were on the upper deck and the spiral stairway down to the exit was too narrow to allow easy egress of the stretcher. The weakened passenger had to walk, heavily supported, down the stairs but eventually managed to get off the plane and on to the ambulance. Our last contact with him was as he drove off with his wife to the local hospital. The airline showed their undying gratitude to us for all our help by giving each of us a small travelling radio clock, and telling us they hoped we would fly Singapore Airlines again . . . We never did hear what became of our patient, but I hope he made a good recovery. Not surprisingly we had no feedback from the other 200 or so passengers as to whether they were pleased or otherwise that we had saved them the inconvenience of landing somewhere in the middle of India.

On another of our holidays we stopped on a cruise in Iceland and while there joined about 30 fellow passengers, nearly all American, on a coach tour of the Country. On the way back to the ship our driver dutifully stopped at a red traffic signal, but the driver of a following juggernaut, loaded with hoisting equipment and concrete, did not think it was necessary. Consequently he smashed into the back of our coach (fortunately made of sturdy material). Although the back of the coach was flattened, the lorry did not actually enter the cabin, but it made a monstrous crashing noise as if the whole bus had exploded under the impact. There was no actual cry of "Is there a doctor present?" but I felt that I had a duty to take some action, or at least to check that no human damage had occurred. In addition, my wife who was sitting next to me, very quickly began jabbing me in the ribs and saying, "Do something", in the way doctors' wives are prone to do. I spoke up: "I'm a doctor, is anyone hurt?" Complete silence greeted the invitation and I sat back reassured. Then an American voice spoke up. "I'm an attorney," he said, "is there anything I can do?" Thirty voices spoke as one. "I think I may have suffered a whiplash injury – can I have your card?"

The last episode I want to relate occurred while we were in the Far East on another cruise. It ended in Tokyo, where we spent three days before flying home. We had arranged to go on a tour of the city and were sitting in the bus in the grounds of the hotel waiting to depart when a frenzied waiter from the hotel came running up to the bus calling, "Is there a doctor on the bus?" With my wife sitting next to me and some of our fellow passengers knowing who I was, there was no escaping into anonymity. I reluctantly revealed myself, realising that I was unlikely to find the bus still waiting by the time I returned. Tokyo would be a no-no.

On returning to the reception hall of the hotel I saw a small group of people standing doing nothing but creating an obstacle to a clear view of the patient. A stern command to "stand aside and let the doctor in" led to them opening up and it was immediately obvious that the cause of the alarm was a young baby of no more than 10 months of age, lying supine across her mother's lap, unconscious and fitting badly. Fortunately this was not a situation in which medical equipment was required and I rapidly managed to lay the baby in the resuscitation position and, on absorbing the brief history that she had been ill with a fever over the past few days, concluded that the most likely diagnosis was fever convulsion. I reassured her mother that although very frightening, the fit would pass, but while someone called for an ambulance it would be wise to cool the baby down by taking off some of the many layers of clothing and blanket covering the child. By the time the ambulance did arrive, the fit had passed off and the baby was reassuringly crying. I later heard that the child then developed a rash and was diagnosed with measles; she made a full recovery. I returned to where I had left the bus expecting it to have gone on its way, but to my delight the passengers had made the driver wait for me, and being mostly American, I was greeted by the sound of applause. I was the hero for the rest of the morning: a very satisfying experience, which was further increased when the grateful parents, who turned out to be on holiday from Hong Kong, presented me with a small piece of pottery in recognition of my help. My ego was further inflated a few months later when I received at home a card from Hong Kong, inside of which was the news that the baby was well and had reached her first birthday.

Compared with some of the stories that one reads in the press, such as the anaesthetist who used a coat hanger to keep someone alive while flying on a plane, my examples may appear rather puny, but each occasion has remained vivid in my memory. You never know what might happen when you hear the call.

CHAPTER XXIV

Honours Even

I have never met Helen Mirren, the famous actor who has played numerous Queens on television, radio, stage and films. However, I have been introduced and met our present Queen on more than one occasion, one of which was extra special.

My first two meetings with her were both at St Bartholomew's Hospital, once when I was on the management committee and she visited the hospital. On that occasion it was only a shake of the hand and no words were passed. The second occasion was more personal. She was visiting the academic departments of the hospital where we had recently set up the department of general practice, the first time that St Bartholomew's had a recognised academic department for the teaching of general practice. It was decided that the Queen would visit our department as part of her tour of the hospital and we would arrange a display to demonstrate the type of work we were doing. We thought it a good idea to demonstrate a role-playing session, which we were still experimenting with as a tool for teaching.

The day of her visit arrived; we were dressed in our academic gowns looking very smart and feeling very distinguished. She arrived in the department with a retinue that included the Duke of Gloucester and took her seat on the chair provided, while we stood around her ready to answer any questions. I believe she was meant to stay about five or ten minutes, but she apparently became very interested and stayed at least half an hour. I was most impressed with her understanding of how general practice worked and the intelligent questions she asked. After all, it cannot be very often that she has sat in a doctor's waiting room in order to be seen.

In November 1991 I received notification of the possibility of being included in the New Year Honours of that year. This came in the first instance as a letter from 10 Downing Street marked "strictly private and confidential", but anyone that knows how our house works will recognise this as a signal for Pearl, my wife, to open it, which she duly did and was therefore the first recipient of the news. For me, it was one of those 'where were you when...' moments that you remember for the rest of your life. I was in the bath, but the excitement and surprise was undiminished in any way.

I still have the letter and have re-examined its contents. It came from the Principal Private Secretary to the Prime Minister, John Major. At this stage I was being informed, in strict confidence, that he had it in mind to submit my name to the Queen with a recommendation "that Her Majesty may be graciously pleased to approve that you be appointed a Member of the Order of the British Empire". There were still several hurdles to be crossed, the first being that I would agree to accept the Honour. Following this the Prime Minister would have to activate what he only had, at this stage, "in his mind to submit". Finally, the Queen herself would have to approve and only then would my name be recorded in the published New Year Honours list. I was finally warned that I would receive no further communication before publication of the list. Having successfully jumped all the hurdles, I was privileged and honoured to appear in the list on 31 December 1991 and could be addressed as James Carne MBE.

"Order of the British Empire" is an anachronism, as we no longer have an empire; perhaps it should be changed to "Order of the British Commonwealth", but it is unlikely that the traditionalists will allow this to happen. I, and I suspect most others who are included in the Order, will agree with Shakespeare that "a rose by any other name will smell as sweet" and we remain honoured to have been included at whichever level we have been appointed.

The next communication came in January 1992 from St James's Palace, informing me that the investiture would take place on 5 March. Full instructions were included and I was invited to take up to three guests if they included my wife and two daughters. I was asked to indicate if any guest would need special arrangements made. As the proposed date was within two weeks of my younger daughter's expected date of delivery for her second child, I requested a seat for her if this was not already automatically provided. The two months between notification and investiture were spent in great trepidation and planning suitable attire for us all but work continued as normal.

The great day eventually became a reality. I had arranged a chauffeur-driven car to transport us to Buckingham Palace and, it being such a special occasion, thought it appropriate to use a one-man firm to whom we had been introduced a few years previously. He was a man in his 60s who had retired from a very prestigious position in the commercial world. Wanting to continue being active he decided to combine this wish with his love of driving, and offered himself and his car for hire. He played the part to perfection. Smart voice, chauffer's uniform, and old-fashioned courtesies such as opening the door for the passenger. I thought he would be suitably impressed by the consignment of taking his passenger to Buckingham Palace to receive an MBE. My pride was somewhat shattered when we arrived and I was trying to tell him the instructions I had received about parking. He listened patiently for a short time and then turned to me and said ever so politely, "Yes, I know. I was there a few years ago, to receive my OBE", with the emphasis firmly on the 'O'.

On entering the palace, I was separated from my family as they were led off to the investiture hall where seats were provided as in a theatre and a band from a Guards regiment played music to entertain them. I was directed to a magnificent waiting area to join all the other recipients of Honours on that day. We in turn had been separated into groups depending on the Honour we had been awarded. On entering the room I was, to my surprise, greeted by name by a charming young lady. I was even more surprised when she asked, "And how is your daughter, Doctor Carne?" In my confusion I replied, "Oh, do you know Jo or Debbie?" She said, "I don't, but you told us one of your daughters is expecting a baby very soon." I remain amazed at the efficiency in this country with which formal affairs are arranged, even at the highest level.

The actual investiture was filmed and I have had the original tape converted to DVD. It reinforces the happy and proud memories I have of a wonderful day. I am often asked if the Queen actually speaks to you when she hands over the medal. In my case she asked where I was in practice, but after that I was overcome by the occasion and do not remember how the rest of the conversation went. I was just about in a fit state to remember that when she extends her hand to shake yours, the interview is at end. A quick bob of the head, right turn and a short walk to a uniformed gentleman at a table to whom you return your valued medal, with his reassurance that it will be returned after it has been boxed. We rounded off a wonderful day by having the rest of the immediate family join us for lunch at the Ritz Hotel.

EPILOGUE

It is now five years since I started recalling the episodes recorded in this book. Number three grandson, Alex, helped me set it up and now, number one grandson, Tom, with the help of Sophie his wife (our honorary granddaughter number one), have edited it with great diligence. It is ready for the publisher and the last opportunity for changes has arrived. In the terms of the first chapter, the sandwich has been made and is ready for the eating. I hear a voice saying "not a sandwich, but a hamburger: what about the garnish?" I reply that I prefer my hamburger plain and would rather not add anything, but leave the memories and episodes recorded here unchanged. Indeed, nothing of great importance has happened. Nothing, that is, that is worth recording, or maybe things have been forgotten or felt to be of less importance as one has advanced from the vintage years to the veteran years. An advantage of old age is that things seem less important, but the accompanying disadvantage is that life is not quite as much fun.

Having written this, within a few hours I had an experience that equals any I have recorded already, so must be added. Pearl and I were walking towards the bus stop at Golders Green Station and the rain was intensifying. We were dressed smartly in dark clothes, as one does when visiting the doctor, and the lure of the taxi rank was too tempting to ignore. Approaching the front cab, we did not know that many customers had preceded us in order to travel to the nearby crematorium. On arrival at the cab, the driver lowered the window and before I could say a word, said "I know, you want to get to the crematorium." "Not yet, I hope," was my spontaneous reply before the irony of the situation struck home. This was the ultimate in feeling old: a taxi driver wanting to take you prematurely to your burial ground. He remained oblivious to what he had just said, and presumably in an effort to be helpful after we had settled down in the back seats, he asked if we were hot enough "or do you want me to put the heat up a bit?" He must have thought we had already arrived at the crematorium!

I remain privileged to continue a happy life together with Pearl, my companion and wife for the past 68 years. We consider ourselves to be fit, but it is difficult to convince BUPA this is so as they relentlessly, year by year, put up our subscriptions "because of our age". We have noticed that we are in danger of being charged overweight on our luggage when we fly to our holiday destination, because of the pills we have to take with us. I blame this on the pharmaceutical industry who keep finding new remedies to keep us fit, but in spite of the aches and pains and other inevitable maladies associated with age, we really do enjoy a contented life. To paraphrase Stephen Sondheim, "We are still here."

I managed to continue carrying out expert witness work for a further ten years after officially retiring, but in the end the realisation that the legal profession had cottoned on to my age and found it too easy to point out (some might say humiliate) to the expert who they were cross examining that he was past being an expert in anything, let alone the complicated subject of medicine, led me to make the inevitable decision to retire fully from medical work. However, although I have retired from active medical work, I have found new-awakened interest in the Retired Fellows Society of the Royal Society of Medicine and am an enthusiastic recipient of their lectures and meetings. I have also been honoured to be elected a Council Member and act as honorary treasurer. I have also increased my number of attendances at The Medical Society of London, the oldest medical society in London having been founded in 1773. It is of interest that the now world renowned and prestigious Royal Society of Medicine was started as an off-shoot of the Medical Society of London, when a group of its Fellows found it impossible to oust their President of twenty one years, a Dr James Sims, in the final years of the 1700's and started their own Society, which, like Topsy, grew and grew. I note from the annual archives of the London Medical Society that I am number three in the list of current Fellows in order of being elected to the Society. However, I know that number one died many years ago, but his name has not yet been removed. That really makes me feel old.

I have decided against adding a relish to my hamburger sandwich, but I will have one last rant. A few years ago the General Medical Council (GMC), with whom you have to be registered in order to practice medicine and prescribe drugs, and for which an annual fee is payable, decided that instead of allowing doctors who had retired from practice to remain on the register without further charge, they should be made to pay a reduced annual fee for the privilege. Many retired doctors decided that it was time to also retire from being registered, and thus save the cost. Others, of whom I am one, feel that registration is a privilege one has earned through years of hard work and study. I liken registration with the GMC with the baton a Field Marshall has earned, and it should not have to be given up merely for the saving of a few pounds. Other Societies and Associations have kept up the tradition of honorary, free membership and the excuse that the GMC had been given legal advice that failure to charge for registration would be unfair to younger practitioners who had to pay, seems spurious in my opinion. I intend to remain registered, pay the fee as long as I can afford it, and retain my dignity. If at some time in the future, the GMC judge me as unfit to be able to continue to practice, I will retire, but until then, I shall continue to carry my baton under my arm. It also means that if a member of my immediate family needs an emergency prescription I will be able to supply it, and if I wish to give professional advice, I am able to do so.

Before concluding I would like to thank all those in the book who are recognisable. To those who have unknowingly provided fodder for some of the episodes described, I repeat that I have made every effort to keep them unrecognisable, and can reassure anyone that thinks they recognise themselves, that it was definitely someone else.

END

ACKNOWLEDGEMENTS

The enjoyment I have had in compiling this book would have been just hard work if it had not been for several people who helped me, in their various ways, to complete the journey.

First my wife, Pearl, and daughters, Joanna Lamont and Debbie Dotsch, for their patience and unique gift of making me feel important, and giving me the confidence to complete the work. My grandson, Tom Lamont, and his wife, Sophie Elmhirst, for casting their professional eyes over the final draft and correcting my numerous grammatical mistakes and excesses. My grandsons, Matt Lamont and Alex and Ollie Dotsch for putting up with my frequent computer problems and nearly always finding a solution. Cleo, my first great grandchild who arrived just in time to be included in this volume.

I would like to thank all my partners and practice staff with whom I worked during the 41 years I remained in general practice. From the single-handed practice I joined in 1957 until my retirement from the large group practice it had grown into by 1998, these were many and varied, but all provided loyalty and support and it is a matter of great pride that many remain in the practice 15 years after I left it.

I also acknowledge the many thousands of patients with whom I came into contact, and whose lives were so often intimately entwined with my own, and especially those who have, anonymously and unrecognised, contributed to some of the anecdotes related in my book.

The editor of the Journal of the Retired Fellows of the Royal Society of Medicine, Richard Lansdown, who has allowed me to reproduce some of the anecdotes that have already been published in the Journal.

The publishers, Grosvenor House Publishing who have helped guide me through the intricacies of bringing my book into print.

And, finally, I would like to acknowledge the successive governments, without whose constant changing of the NHS rules, life would not have been nearly so interesting.

James Carne

Word Count: 73,468.

Lightning Source UK Ltd.
Milton Keynes UK
UKOW03n0847110514

231462UK00002B/13/P